IN YOUR OWN TIME

a guide for patients and their carers facing a last illness at home

Elizabeth Lee

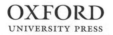

OXFORD
UNIVERSITY PRESS

OXFORD

UNIVERSITY PRESS

Great Clarendon Street, Oxford OX2 6DP

Oxford University Press is a department of the University of Oxford.
It furthers the University's objective of excellence in research, scholarship,
and education by publishing worldwide in

Oxford   New York

Auckland   Bangkok   Buenos Aires   Cape Town   Chennai
Dar es Salaam   Delhi   Hong Kong   Istanbul   Karachi   Kolkata
Kuala Lumpur   Madrid   Melbourne   Mexico City   Mumbai
Nairobi   São Paulo   Shanghai   Taipei   Tokyo   Toronto

and an associated company in Berlin

Oxford is a registered trade mark of Oxford University Press
in the UK and in certain other countries

Published in the United States
by Oxford University Press Inc., New York

© Elizabeth Lee, 2002

A catalogue record for this title is available from the British Library

Library of Congress Cataloging in Publication Data

(Data available)

ISBN 0 19 850975 8 (Pbk)

10 9 8 7 6 5 4 3 2 1

Typeset by Cepha Imaging Pvt Ltd

Printed in Great Britain
on acid-free paper by Biddles Ltd, Guildford & King's Lynn

Contents

Acknowledgements ix

Introduction xi

CHAPTER ONE

Facing Bad News 1

Approaching death 3
• *How will you know?*

Getting bad news 6
• *How long have I got?* • *Hope*
• *What to do with bad news*

Treatment 11
• *The internet* • *Treatment
decisions* • *Complementary
therapy* • *Counselling*

Getting practical help 20
• *Statutory services* • *Charities
and self-help groups*

Thinking ahead 25
• *Becoming a carer* • *Home or
hospital*

CHAPTER TWO

At Home 29

Community medical care 30
• *The key worker* • *The district
nurse* • *The general practitioner*

Specialists involved in care
at home 51
• *The home care specialist
nurse* • *Hospice at home*

• *Other specialist nurses*
• *Specialist doctors* • *Other sources of support*

What can go wrong   **61**

Summary   **66**

CHAPTER THREE
....
Hospital, Hospice or Home?   **67**

Hospital care   **68**
• *Why hospital?* • *Which hospital?*
• *Choosing your hospital* • *Other patients* • *Patients' relationships with staff* • *Relationships between staff and carers* • *Patients' feelings*
• *How to make a decision*

The hospice and palliative care services   **94**
• *How do you feel about hospices?*
• *Why choose a hospice?* • *Referrals to hospital and hospice*

CHAPTER FOUR
....
Patients and Carers   **107**

Patients' feelings   **108**
• *Denial* • *Anger* • *Bargaining*
• *Depression* • *Acceptance*
• *Where are you?* • *Positive experiences*

Preoccupying problems   **118**
• *Your dependants* • *Unfinished business* • *Legal matters*

Shared concerns of patient and carer   **133**
• *Practical matters* • *The funeral*
• *Your relationship* • *Family matters*

Contents

Carers' concerns   142
• *Good feelings* • *Angry feelings*
• *Selfish feelings* • *Anxiety*
• *Practical concerns*

CHAPTER FIVE

Common Symptoms and Their
Treatment   157

Talking about your symptoms   157
• *What influences our symptoms?*

Anxiety   160

Sleeplessness   163

Depression   166

Constipation   167

Bed sores   171

Mouth care   174

Pain   175
• *Drug treatment* • *Pain requiring
special treatment*

Nausea and vomiting   185

Loss of appetite   188

Difficulty breathing   190
• *Anxiety and fear* • *Treatment*

Loss of bladder control   194

Loss of bowel control   197

Confusion   198

Cannabis   203

Contents

CHAPTER SIX
....
Last Days   **205**

• *Saying goodbye* • *Distress*
• *Last hours* • *Letting go*

APPENDICES
....
**Appendix 1: What to do After
a Death**   **217**

**Appendix 2: Checklist of Statutory
Benefits**   **219**

**Appendix 3: Useful Sources of
Information and Support**   **223**
• *General* • *Organizations for
patients with cancer* • *Other
specific organizations*
• *Complementary medicine*
• *Bereavement services*

**Appendix 4: Recommended
Reading**   **241**

Index   **243**

Acknowledgements

I would like to acknowledge and thank the following people who have allowed me to write about their personal experience of illness, whether it be their own or that of a loved one: Arthur Brown, Sacha Craddock, Lorna Durkin, Audrey Jenkins, Diana Millbank, Maryanne Moore, Mary Rapps, Joan Welsh, Rosemary Lunn, Clive and Sarah Frankish, and Gill Walkey.

I have particularly valued the advice and guidance of the following district nursing sisters and community nurses: Nikki Jordan, Chris Carr, Jean Culverwell, Carol Gendle, Jill Briggs and Penny Roberts, and the specialist nurses Sue Thomas, Community Health Adviser, Royal College of Nursing and Nikki Spencer, Marie Curie Organizer. I would especially like to thank Ellen Richardson, whose close cooperation during the early stages of writing this book helped shape it and taught me to understand and value the expertise and sensitivity of many working in the field of palliative care medicine. Thanks also to Dr William M. O'Neill; to Dr R. Jones; to Dr David Seamark of The Institute of General Practice, Exeter University; to David Towers, Medical Social Worker; and to Hillary Holman, tutor, St Peter's Hospice for the time they spent talking to me.

I am particularly grateful to the Reverend Ian Hoskins for the two case histories that he has contributed to the book.

Many people read and offered advice on the text and I am very grateful to them all but would especially like to thank my husband Dr David Kessler and my parents Dr Alan Lee and Dr Patricia Thompson for their invaluable advice born out of many years of experience in listening to and caring for patients. Thanks also to Beth Kessler for her wisdom and her support and to my editor Judy Warren for the sensitivity with which she has edited this book and Martin Baum at Oxford University Press.

My thanks to Faber & Faber for permission to quote from Dennis Potter's *Seeing the Blossom* in Chapter 4.

Introduction

This is a book for patients who are facing a final illness and for those who are caring for them at home. It has two main purposes: to give information about what help and support is available and ways of getting access to it, and to describe what choices are open to you so that you can get the kind of care you want.

You may not feel that you have the strength, the time or the desire to read a book at such a time. You may feel overwhelmed by all the changes you are going through, and if this is so you may like to ask a friend or member of your family to read it for you. They can use the information in the book to make sure that you are offered the best quality of life in the time that is left to you.

A lot has changed in the last twenty years, in part due to technological developments, and many symptoms can now be treated as effectively at home as in hospital. The work of the district nurse and general practitioner (GP) is complemented by specialist nurses expert in caring for people who are dying. Another significant change is that nurses and GPs are now taught to look after patients holistically, acknowledging that psychological, spiritual and social factors are inextricably bound up with our feelings of well-being. Social workers, clergy of all faiths, practitioners of complementary medicine and many others are there to help you and your family.

When I worked as a GP in a deprived inner city practice in London I saw that some patients had access to all kinds of support while others had very little help at all. The patients who had good support usually had an advocate—someone who was determined to fight for the help they needed, and who could effectively communicate those needs to the various professionals involved. Some patients acted as their own advocate. Then I moved to Bristol and worked in a practice that served a cohesive community. Families lived near to each other and there was tremendous support for patients who became ill. The district nurses and GPs knew their patients well and it was a great pleasure to see the high standard of care they gave to those who were dying.

I believe that everyone should have access to this level of care and in this book I explain clearly and simply what I consider to be an acceptable standard of good care. If your care is inadequate you should feel confident to demand that it improves, and improves now, not next month or next year. Often you just need to ask, but you need to know what to ask for. Sometimes you need to take more drastic steps.

When you are dying you and your family face difficult decisions about the kind of care you want and where you want to receive it—whether, for example, you want to be at home, in hospital or in a hospice. To make the right decisions you need to understand what your options are, find out what choices you may have. I have tried throughout to be realistic so as not to mislead people. There is no point choosing to be cared for in a community hospital if there isn't one near you. Choices vary from place to place and from illness to illness, and I give straightforward guidance about how to find out what choices are available to you.

Death and what lies beyond remains a mystery to me, as it did to Robert Frost who wrote:

There may be much or little beyond the grave,
The strong are saying nothing till they see.[1]

But we know from many, many first-hand accounts what the process of dying can be like. Throughout this book there are personal accounts from people who have walked this road before you. They are all very different but nevertheless a commonality of experience is revealed in them. Perhaps by sharing them you will feel less alone. By reading about the road others have taken, the problems they have met and the solutions they have found, I hope you will feel more prepared to face the difficult days and months that lie ahead.

[1]*Extract from 'The Strong are Saying Nothing' from The Poetry of Robert Frost, edited by Edward Connery Lathem, the Estate of Robert Frost and Jonathan Cape as publisher. Used by permission of The Random House Group Limited.*

For David, Georgia and Joe

1
Facing Bad News

No one ever tells us what it is like to die, it is a secret known only to the dying. I have done my best to listen to dying patients and their carers, to hear what they are saying and to understand how they are feeling. What I have learnt is that there are as many ways of facing death as there are individuals in this world.

Over the years I have witnessed many people die. What is a 'good death'? The quick death afforded by a massive heart attack has much to recommend it. Yet it is the patients who have the chance to get to know death, who have the courage to look him in the eye and finally not to feel afraid, who have set their affairs in order, have said goodbye and made their peace with life, these are the deaths that I think of as 'good'. But I recognize that for many people this path towards a graceful acceptance is the antithesis of everything they feel. They have no intention of making the best of a bad job. They go out angry and fighting. As a doctor or a carer these are much more difficult deaths to live with—in fact they can be hell for all concerned. Slowly, however, I have come to recognize that there is an uncompromising honesty in the way such people express their agony, their sadness, their anger, in the way they refuse to capitulate and insist, it seems, on behaving 'badly'. It is their way of dying and it is OK. There is no right or wrong way, no good or bad way to die.

This book takes you through the choices that exist in the current system of medical care, to help you decide on the kind of care you want and where you receive it. Through knowing what help is available and the standards of good care you should expect, you and your carer will be able to make properly informed decisions. I also talk about the feelings that both patients and carers experience when they are coming to terms with a final illness. I hope the book will help you to face death in your own way.

The Irish have a saying: 'twenty years a growing, twenty years a blooming, twenty years declining, twenty years a dying'. It is a recognition of the ever-turning cycle of life, particularly heartening in that it gives us a decade more than the commonly quoted three score years and ten. More than half the population of the western world now live to be older than seventy-five. Recently an old lady said to me with evident satisfaction 'I've had a good innings, doctor.' This familiar cricketing metaphor rings true; we can't all hope to hit a century, but a good innings of seventy or eighty is something to be proud of. Rather different from the batsman bowled out in the teens before he had got his eye in. Patients who become terminally ill when they are young are often described as having an 'interrupted biography'. Their feelings, those of their family and friends, and indeed of society as a whole, will clearly be quite different from the man or woman who has reached their eighth decade.

Approaching death

Every child knows that we all die and yet we continue to live as if we were immortal. When does someone become terminally ill? It is a question that demands an answer. Only when a patient has faced the probability of his own death can he start the work—emotional and practical—that will help him die more peacefully. This does not mean that all hope has been abandoned. Maintaining hope is part of the human condition and can coexist with an awareness of death. Recognition that someone is terminally ill, however, means that many of the support systems within our society can spring into action, offering help to him and his carers in all sorts of different ways.

How will you know?

Patients often understand their own bodies and feel a change that is different from any that has gone before. They do not need a doctor to tell them that they are dying. Carers, too, can often know, especially if they have looked after their loved one for a long time.

Case history

Mr Davies was the most genial of eighty year olds. He told me with pride that he had played the bugle in the local school band before the First World War. His wife, who was much younger, was very dedicated to him. When he could no longer go up the road for his regular pint we realized that he was getting ill. A blood test showed anaemia. I came and talked to him about what this might imply but he chose not to go up to the hospital for any other tests, nor would he have any truck

---

with specialists. He was sitting up in his chair chatting as usual when I left. Two days later I was surprised to find that his wife was making a bed downstairs for him. She told me her husband was dying and that she intended to nurse him there in the front room. He died four days later. His wife had been right. She did not need tests or medical training, she knew enough by knowing the patient.

Of course people can be wrong. One lunchtime I was boiling some potatoes when the phone rang and I was asked to attend an old Bangladeshi woman. 'Can I come in half an hour?' I asked optimistically, hoping to save the potatoes. 'No, please come straight away, she is dying.' I rushed round to find the whole extended family gathered around the bed. The little frail old woman had summoned them all to be with her at the moment of her death, as is the Muslim custom. I knelt down and began to examine her, performing my role confidently in front of the assembled family, expecting to confirm their worst fears. But to my discomfort I could find nothing wrong. Surely my patient knew something that I didn't? I took courage and said, 'I do not think you are dying just at the moment' and left requesting I be called immediately if her condition changed. She did live; she had misread the signs of her impending death.

Patients with cancer

The diagnosis of cancer can be a devastating blow, yet with many cancers the initial diagnosis is not a diagnosis of terminal illness. Perhaps it is only when the disease is spreading that we begin to think of death as the final outcome. The initial diagnosis of cancer is therefore like a warning shot, jolting you, forcing you to recognize the possibility of your own mortality. Some people find this jolt alters their perception of life in a profound way. Time becomes more precious, values that for years have been unthinkingly accepted are re-examined. Perhaps you feel a need for change; perhaps you wish to be more true to yourself. Good can come out of what has happened to you.

For some cancers it is different. No one knows how long you have to live, and with treatment you can certainly be made to feel better, but there is no cure. You may have been plunged straight from good health into a terminal illness and this can be devastating. It will take time for you to grasp what has happened to you and begin to accept it.

In Chapter 4 the way people feel when they are facing death is examined in some detail.

Patients with other conditions

Some patients are ill for many years. The series of losses that are part and parcel of dying creep up gradually in these patients. Usually there comes a time when doctors can say 'This patient is going to die soon.' The trouble is that they can be very bad at saying this. Because the downward path slopes so gradually they forget that it ever reaches an end. Of course it does, and all concerned, doctor, patient, carer, should look out for that end, anticipate it, and plan for it.

> **Case history**
> John was a young man who died of multiple sclerosis at twenty-nine. He was cared for at home by his family.

Towards the end he could no longer talk or do anything for himself. Up until then he had not been in pain, but suddenly he appeared to be uncomfortable, and his GP and family together decided to start him on morphine. At this moment they formally recognized that he was dying, but there was now no opportunity to talk to him. It was too late. They should have talked to him about dying long before he lost the power of speech. He must have known that he was dying, must have feared it, but nobody was ready to hear him.

Getting bad news

Most people are given bad news by their doctor. This interview can have a profound effect on how you come to terms with your future. Breaking bad news is very difficult, and even experienced doctors have to steel themselves to do it. Some are good at it, some are poor, most fall somewhere in between. Ideally bad news should be broken to you gently, in a private place where there is no possibility of being disturbed. Your partner or a close friend should either be present or nearby, and plenty of time should be set aside for you to ask any questions. You will certainly think of more questions later, after you have had time to absorb some of the shock, and so a further appointment may be arranged.

If this most difficult of meetings was handled sensitively and honestly you may feel ready to explore what you can now do to help yourself, armed with a real understanding of what is going to happen to you. Although the possibility of a cure may not have been held out to you, you should not feel totally abandoned. There being no known cure for your disease is not the same as saying 'there is nothing more that can be done for you'. This book is all about what can be done for you from this point onwards.

If bad news was broken to you badly you will feel understandably angry and resentful towards the person responsible. No one can turn the clock back and run the scene again, no one can undo what has happened. If you have had bad news ineptly broken you may want to tell that person how you feel. It may even afford them the chance to understand what went wrong and change the way they work in future. Talk to them about it or, if it is easier, write. The first verse of 'A Poison Tree', from William Blake's *Songs of Experience* expresses with beautiful simplicity the effect of anger that remains unexpressed.

I was angry with my friend:
I told my wrath, my wrath did end.
I was angry with my foe:
I told it not, my wrath did grow.

How long have I got?

This is the question that everyone asks and no one answers. The unwritten code of practice among doctors is to reply, 'I would love to give you an answer but the truth is that no one knows.' Of course no one knows, but it is a singularly unhelpful response. I think all doctors can give some idea, and if you need an answer to this question you should encourage them to throw caution to the wind and make a best guess. Those that stubbornly refuse to can often be pinned down by your asking 'If it was *your* mother who was ill like this, how long would you guess?'

But remember it will be a guess and, where some diseases are concerned, very imprecise. For example, I had two patients that died of multiple sclerosis in the same month. One had lived with her illness for fifty years, the other had died within ten.

Some people are near death for months or years and because their illness does not follow a natural and predictable progression it is impossible to say when they will die, though it is possible to predict how. Chronic respiratory failure is the commonest example. A patient may live with this condition for some years yet it is likely that flu or a chest infection will be the eventual cause of death.

Sometimes the patient is ahead of the doctor. A friend of mine told me this story about his father. It was one of his father's last good jokes. Mr Burrows developed fluid on the lung and so he was sent for a chest X-ray. When he went to the hospital for the result he saw a pleasant Egyptian doctor who told him that he had bad news. The doctor put the X-ray up on a screen and indicated the white shadow of a lung cancer. 'I suppose that's curtains then,' said Mr Burrows. 'Oh no, no,' said the doctor in alarm, waving his hand at the shadow, 'this is not the curtains Mr Burrows.'

Hope

Very rarely do people 'turn their face to the wall' after being given bad news. Usually they struggle with and against it, and eventually gain the strength and the courage to live with the knowledge of their own death. During this struggle they are sustained by hope, hope which humans should never abandon. It may be hope of a cure, realistic or unrealistic, or hope that some research is about to produce a new drug that will give many more years of life. When people know that they are dying the things they hope for change. You may hope to see one more spring, to complete an important piece of work, or to hold your grandchild in your arms.

The Ancient Greeks illustrated the power of hope in the story of Pandora's box, their myth of the fall. Pandora was instructed never to open the box that the gods had given to her husband as a wedding present. Eventually her curiosity got the better of her. As she turned the key, intending just to peep inside, the lid flew open and all the evils of the world surged out: disease, cruelty, pain, hatred, poverty, disappointment, jealousy, war and death. In horror she slammed the box closed, but a little voice inside called out 'Pandora, do not shut me in, for without me you will not be able to bear all the unhappiness that you have turned loose.' So Pandora lifted the lid and out fluttered hope. As it passed out into the world a watery sun broke through the raging storm and howling wind. Prometheus chained for eternity to the side of a cliff, pecked at all day long by eagles, felt hope enter his heart, hope that one day he would be set free.

What to do with bad news

It is difficult for experienced doctors to break bad news and they have lots of practice. It is much more difficult for patients and carers who have to decide what to do with the news. Who are you going to tell, and how are you going to tell them? There will be family, friends, neighbours, workmates. The list can be long and the task daunting. If you are a couple it may be easier to do the telling together. You will need privacy (take the telephone off the hook) and protected time when no one has to rush off.

I find I break bad news badly when I have not prepared myself and it all spills out too fast. I do better if I have rehearsed the scene in my head beforehand. Timing is very important, and some people like to sit on the news for a little while before they feel ready to share it.

> **Case history**
>
> Mrs Williams had to go into hospital for an operation to confirm what was suspected to be cancer of the bowel. For weeks she and her husband had been looking forward to having their little grandson for the weekend while his parents went away. They knew their daughter would not go once she learned about the operation. They did not want to spoil her trip and also they desperately wanted the pleasure of their grandson. So they planned to tell her on the Sunday night when she came back. This they did and Mrs Williams went into hospital the next day.

In what order are you going to tell people? People are very sensitive about this sort of thing and it is worth thinking about who will be upset if they hear the news via a third party. If telling is too difficult you can ask for help. Your doctor will help you tell close family if you ask. Many people delegate the job to a friend or relative and this saves going over and over the facts with lots of people. It also protects you from some of the distress that the news provokes.

Telling children is particularly difficult and many families balk at the idea, believing that the children are too young to understand or to cope with the information. All the evidence suggests that children can't really be protected in this way. Often the effect of these well-meaning intentions is to isolate children and increase their loneliness. All children say that regardless of whether they were told or not they knew something was wrong. Seeing their mother or father upset or ill made them feel lonely and afraid, and some felt that they were not allowed to ask questions. Just because they do not ask does not mean that children do not want to know. If they understand how serious the illness is they can have the opportunity to help and to get closer to their parent.

If telling your children is too difficult you may need someone to help you. Hospice staff can be experienced at talking to children about their feelings and fears. Your GP, district or school nurse, social worker or priest may all be able to ease your burden by sharing some of the 'telling'. After the telling comes the listening—listening to the child's fears, answering questions, allowing them to express pain. Children often worry that they are responsible for a parent's illness or death, and it is only by talking to them that these fantasies can be revealed. And just like everyone else, children sometimes need permission to forget about illness, to laugh, to play, to get on with normal life.

There are several booklets that deal with the problems of telling children. You can find them at your local hospice.

Treatment

Every patient needs to be confident that they have had the best treatment that is available. Medical advances are always being reported, it seems, and you need to be certain that the doctors looking after you are right up to date.

How do you do this? For most people it is easy. They trust their GP and their specialist to be acting in their best interest. It is clear that they are getting the same treatment as other patients they know. Everything they read or hear confirms that they are being treated properly.

But what if you find another patient who is receiving different treatment or has been referred to a specialist hospital when you have not? Or you read in a magazine about a new treatment being pioneered somewhere else? Bear in mind that you cannot easily compare yourself with another patient. There are almost certainly different factors operating in each case that affect the very complicated treatment decisions that have been made. Nevertheless, if you have a whiff of anxiety about your treatment you need to ask someone to explain why your treatment decisions were taken. Your specialist is probably the best person to ask. Alternatively try your GP.

If you want more information or are worried that you are getting a parochial view of the problem, there are several sources of information for you to tap. Information about treatment for all types of cancer is provided by a number of groups. In Scotland, for example, Tak Tent gives information and emotional support to cancer patients. CancerLink is a central publishing and information resource for patients and families. The National AIDS Helpline provides information and telephone counselling for patients with AIDS. There is the Motor Neurone Disease Association, the Multiple Sclerosis Society, the Parkinson's Disease Society and so on. Each organization should have someone who can talk to you about acceptable standards of treatment. Details of some national organizations are given in Appendix 3, pp. 223–240. You can look others up in the telephone directory or telephone NHS Direct who will research local resources for you.

The internet

Many people are using the internet as a source both of information and of support. Aside from email, looking for medical information is now the commonest use of the web. A very good place to start if you have cancer is the BACUP website which provides extensive information on all aspects of living with cancer. You will find it at www.cancerbacup.org.uk. Other illnesses that have national or local support groups can also be found on the web and are certainly worth exploring. If you are unable to get out and about because of your illness or because you are a full-time carer, the internet may be a particularly useful tool.

Professional organizations can be helpful, but sometimes better still are email groups. For example, if you have breast cancer you may like to 'talk' to other women with breast cancer by joining an email group. There are groups for all kinds of illness for patients, carers and professionals. So, for example, if your mother has breast cancer there will probably be a specific group for children of women with breast cancer. One of the best informed patients I have ever met was a man with cancer of the larynx who was a dedicated internet user. In hospital he was offered a choice of two different speaking valves following his laryngectomy. Through his email group he knew that there was a far greater variety available. He argued persuasively for a change in hospital policy, saying 'if I need glasses I don't want a choice of just two pairs and the same is true for my speaking valve.'

Treatment decisions

Once you feel confident that you are being offered the best treatment currently available you will probably find that it is easier to choose what treatment you want. Some treatment will be aimed at curing you, some at giving you symptom relief. There is no doubt that the medical profession's increasing desire to share treatment decisions with patients is right and good. Yet it can create problems. The old-fashioned paternalistic approach relieves both patient and carer of certain responsibilities. A woman with inoperable cancer of the ovary had had three courses of chemotherapy, but the disease was spreading. All that her consultant had left to offer her was a new, experimental drug. With this she had a one in five chance of some remission, of living for a few more months. But her hair would certainly fall out during the treatment. The consultant remarked to me 'I don't think patients should be asked to make a decision like this with an experimental drug. They always say yes, take the chance, but it is often the wrong choice. Really we should be taking it for them.' These difficult questions are discussed further in the section on 'living wills' on p. 129.

If you trust your doctor you can ask her to make the decision for you and if she finds this difficult, say 'Doctor, tell me what would you do if you were me?' You still get to make the decision but the doctor will have helped you by honestly answering your question.

Second opinions

At any stage during treatment it is not uncommon for a patient to want a second opinion, or the opinion of a recognized expert. Ask your GP to arrange this for you. You are entitled to a second opinion on the NHS.

Case history

Mr Licata was an Italian patient who was dying from a rare cancer. He felt that he needed to seek the opinion of an Italian specialist. (It is an interesting cultural observation that people only really trust their own health system.) His family proposed flying him to Rome but clearly he was in no condition to travel. As a compromise his doctors sent a copy of his medical records to the Italian expert who was able to review the case and confirm that his treatment was correct. Nothing would be gained by travelling to Italy. Finally Mr Licata was reassured.

Complementary therapy

There is something relentlessly narrow in the conventional medical approach to illness. Nearly all doctors and nurses instinctively take control of your illness, whether they intend to or not: 'This is your diagnosis, this is how we will treat it for you.' When you ask 'What can I do for myself?' they have no answer. Conventional medicine appears to deny you an active role in the fight against your illness.

Complementary medicine is holistic in that each individual is recognized to be so much more than the sum of his individual parts. It seeks to treat the spiritual, emotional and mental causes of illness which finally affect the body in a physical way. This differs from conventional medicine which is primarily directed towards treating physical symptoms. An individual's relationship with himself, with his environment and with life itself are all equally important—mind, body and spirit are interlocked. Complementary medicine also differs from conventional medicine in the importance it places on natural energy or vitality. Natural energy has many different names. In homeopathy it is called the vital force, in yoga it is *prana*, in shiatsu it is *ki* and in acupuncture it is called *chi*. Holistic practitioners will consider how your energy is being drained, how it is affected by what you eat, how you work, your relationships, your philosophy of life. They try to unblock your energy centres and thus establish a state of balance. This will give you strength to find your own way of coping with your life and your illness.

There are a host of complementary therapies where a patient's participation is central to the treatment, and Britain is a country in which they thrive. Many such therapies are directly descended from ancient traditions; healing, for example, has been practised in Britain for centuries and there continue to be healers working in all parts of the country. Healing is not about miracle cures—it is about holistically healing your spirit, body and mind. Ancient Eastern practices have also flourished here—acupuncture and shiatsu massage, to name but two, have a very real role in the care of sick or dying patients. Homeopaths, osteopaths and chiropractors are widespread and in most areas of the country you will be able to find complementary practitioners.

Why are doctors so worried about holistic practices, why do I myself have reservations? Well, I think doctors have all seen patients who have chased hope from one therapy to another, never finding comfort, and spending a great deal of money on the way. False hope blossoms repeatedly, followed by the dejection of failure. We have all seen patients who have fallen into the hands of charlatans. I once had to admit two teenagers to hospital after their alternative practitioner stopped my conventional treatment for their eczema and replaced it with his own. On closer inspection his 'special ointment' was a heat treatment like Algipan, and those children nearly died from loss of fluid through their inflamed skin.

Doctors do have genuine worries. But their attitude is essentially protectionist. The medical profession demand quantitative scientific verification for therapies that cannot be quantified, and have, until recently, ignored all qualitative research. This is changing, very slowly, and I hope within my working lifetime to see a real respect developing between different practitioners.

I advise my patients to go to a recognized natural health centre where several practitioners work together. They should all be registered, so you can be sure that they are fully trained. If there is no such centre near to you contact the appropriate organization (see p. 236) to get a list of local practitioners.

The next step is to find an alternative therapist who suits you. Make a single appointment to start with so that you can easily change therapist if you don't feel comfortable with that particular one. Instead of selecting an individual therapist, some patients with cancer choose a residential course of therapy. The Bristol Cancer Help Centre is a leading centre for the practice of holistic medicine in Britain. In their warm and caring environment people with cancer and their carers are helped to recover from the impact of diagnosis. They receive healing, counselling, massage and learn visualization techniques that help to illuminate hidden or suppressed feelings. At a week-long residential course patients and carers alike draw particular strength from living and sharing experiences with other people in their situation. The centre also employs several doctors who understand both conventional medical treatments and complementary therapies. Self-help techniques of relaxation, meditation and visualization are taught. Everyone is encouraged to rediscover their sources of creativity. People often find their sense of humour comes back. New values, goals and priorities may emerge as a result of this experience and certainly many people gain new energy, hope and direction. Thoughtful loving care like this enables some patients genuinely to say the unthinkable— that having cancer was the best thing that ever happened to them. Here was a chance to stop and look clearly at their life, to listen to themselves, to hear the inner voice that had been lost for so long under the worries and preoccupations of everyday life.

If only this care were available on the NHS, but sadly it is not. It is expensive to go on a Bristol course. Nevertheless, anyone can telephone or write to find out about the centre and its work and doing so may give you other ideas to follow up. It may feel like a bold step to take but you may find it proves rewarding.

The Bristol Cancer Help Centre focuses a lot of attention on diet. Other complementary therapies do likewise. This gives patients the chance to regain control over a much neglected area of their lives and to 'do something'. Your local natural health centre will almost certainly be able to give you guidance on diet if you are interested.

Relaxation, massage and aromatherapy are all practised extensively with patients and their carers. Many hospices have an aromatherapist. One Macmillan nurse told me how wonderful it was to enter her hospice and be greeted by the scent of essential oils. Patients, visitors and staff all love it. Massage can be given regularly to patients and to carers; anyone can learn to give it. I am certain that by unlocking tensions these techniques can reduce the need for all kinds of conventional drugs. Massage is a very good way of bringing touch and physical contact back into many families who are otherwise inhibited. It can be a simple physical way of expressing love.

Throughout holistic medicine runs the theme of self-responsibility. People are encouraged to take responsibility for their own health and well-being. At a time of crisis, of poor or failing health, this may be too difficult to achieve alone. The role of the therapist is then to help build your natural energy levels to a point where you are lifted out of your fear, anxiety and pain. You regain a sense of control. As the spirit is helped through the healing process, death becomes far easier to accept and face.

Counselling

Naturally this is a time of emotional turmoil. Painful feelings and difficult decisions cannot easily be put aside or ignored. For many it is a time when old and unresolved problems resurface. In order to face the present, these old anxieties and troubles also need to be explored and resolved.

Friends and family may be wonderful at listening and giving support but sometimes they are too close to you to help you to fully *explore* these difficult emotions. A counsellor will also be warm and empathic yet can be more objective than those who know you well. They will provide a safe space for you where all that matters are your feelings. They will not be afraid of your emotional pain.

If you would like to see a counsellor there are several places to seek one out. One option is to pay for private sessions. Alternatively, you may find that a counsellor works in the general practice that you attend and you will be able to see them on the health service. If not, your GP or hospital specialist may be able to refer you to a counsellor at the hospital. A third possibility is to see a counsellor through one of the voluntary organizations. The Terrence Higgins Trust Lighthouse, for example, employs counsellors who work with people whose lives have been affected by HIV and AIDS. Many other voluntary organizations, such as Tak Tent, provide free counselling for specific groups of patients. Check the list of useful sources of support and information at the back of this book for details.

When choosing a counsellor you need to make sure that you find someone who is properly trained and highly skilled. A list of qualified counsellors can be obtained from the British Association for Counselling and Psychotherapy. Some organizations offer a befriending service, which is different from a counselling service. Counselling is also different from the supportive care given by your doctors and nurses. Different kinds of emotional support suit different people and many do not want or need counselling at this time. But for some the safe space and time available in a formal counselling relationship makes an enormous difference to their lives.

Getting practical help

When faced with the prospect of death many people put their heads down and struggle on, never realizing that all kinds of practical help are available if they only knew to ask. It may be difficult for you to think of yourself as someone 'in need', particularly if you have had no contact with social services in the past. You may not yet feel ready to identify yourself in this way. Nevertheless, it is important that you think about help to which you may be entitled—it could make all the difference to you and your family.

Statutory services

Since the introduction of the Community Care Act in 1993, local authorities have been required to carry out co-ordinated assessments of individuals who are in need. In the past needs were not formally assessed but were rather haphazardly guessed at by several different professionals. Under the new act, which is designed to be client-centred, the assessment is co-ordinated by one person, which streamlines the system.

What does this mean to you in reality? It means that you are entitled to ask for an assessment of your needs from social services. Be aware that this will not necessarily include an assessment of the needs and wishes of your carers unless the carer specifically asks for help or is clearly in need of it. The Community Care Act relies on you asking for help. In this way the government hopes to limit the amount of care provided. You can ask for an assessment by contacting your local social services office (the address will be in the phone book). Or someone can contact them for you, for example your carer, a friend, your district or home care nurse, or your hospital social worker.

Once you have asked for an assessment you wait. You should have an assessment within five days of the request being made. Assessment can be made by one of several professionals: in my local social services, most are carried out either by a social worker, a home care organizer or an occupational therapist. These three services collaborate closely and, generally, they try to fit the assessor to your perceived needs. For example, a client who needs advice about financial help or respite care will probably be allocated to the social worker. If the main concern is self-care, help with washing, dressing, shopping, laundry or cleaning, the home care organizer will make the assessment. The occupational therapist will be chosen if physical aids are needed to preserve independent living: hand rails, stair lifts, kitchen aids, for example. They can all get you mobile meals (meals on wheels); they can all identify your need for more nursing support and have the power to arrange it. These are the statutory services, and everyone is entitled to be assessed for them.

Of course this is not a panacea. Resources are as limited as they ever were. There is a complicated matrix into which information from the assessment is fitted in order to determine priorities. Your needs will be provided for according to the available resources. Obviously there is a danger of raising false expectations of help—help which never materializes. The provision of funding to the community is a political hot potato and out of your control. As a client all you can do is ask for an assessment, and make sure that you spell out the needs of you and your carers loud and clear.

If social services are told that a patient is terminally ill they do seem to expedite the assessment and implement its recommendations quickly. Recently a stair lift was installed for one of my patients within two weeks of first contacting them. Usually things do not happen this fast. Any delay in the provision of services is particularly cruel when a client is very ill—any delay may leave the carer exhausted and the patient in hospital. It is tempting to say, 'Oh, I'm coping all right at the moment so I'll leave it for a few weeks', only to find yourself with what would have been an avoidable crisis on your hands. Contact social services early. They are one of the main sources of support for patients who are terminally ill at home.

Financial assistance

Being ill is expensive. Heating bills go up when you are cared for at home, travelling to and from appointments or visiting the hospital costs money. There may be changes in diet where expensive special food is required, or special clothing or extra equipment may be needed. Or you have to employ a home help, perhaps pay for nursery places for children. Nine per cent of patients with cancer even have to move house. All this comes at a time when you are probably also experiencing a loss of income.

Eighty-five per cent of people with cancer do not get any financial assistance. Most are simply not told that it is available. Patients who die of non-malignant diseases fare no better.

Case history

Mr Clark had severe emphysema and spent the last eight years of his life propped up in a chair. He could not go out, he couldn't even go to bed because lying down made his breathlessness intolerable. His wife and daughter cared for him through all those dreadful eight years; his wife was lucky if she got three hours off a week. Two years before he died someone finally told them about the attendance allowance. Although he then claimed it until he died, the family have never managed to backdate the claim for the lost six years. They feel very strongly that patients and carers need to look out for themselves and make sure they claim all to which they are entitled.

If you have had contact with social services you should have been advised about grants and allowances. Charities can also provide a great deal of help. There is a brief checklist in Appendix 2 (p. 219), but for fuller details get the leaflet 'Sick or Disabled' from your local social security office. Better still, if like me you find these things confusing ring the Benefits Enquiry Line on 0800 882200 or visit your local citizens' advice centre and they will help you sort everything out.

Charities and self-help groups

Numerous charitable bodies and self-help groups may provide you with social, financial and emotional support. They operate at a local and national level. You can look them up in the phone book or on the internet, or go to the library where there will be a directory of charities.

What can they do for you? Some offer advice and counselling. At a national level they provide information and literature: the Motor Neurone Disease Association, for example, has an excellent pamphlet about dying and the Parkinson's Disease Society has a quarterly newsletter. These organizations also give a political voice to patients with that disease. If you have a local branch, particularly if it is an active one, you may find a pool of support from fellow sufferers or carers. Another great advantage of a local group is that they know what services are available to you. They provide social functions and support groups for both carers and sufferers and 'visiting friends'. One of my patients was very active in her local group. There is a lovely set of photographs of her taken on day trips all over London, smiling in the summer sunshine on Hampstead Heath, visiting Hampton Court. There is even a picture taken around 1965 by a swimming pool in a Spanish hotel. Rose was in a wheelchair all this time and the trips were only possible with the help of the local group who provided transport.

Other people with similar problems to your own can be a mine of information. You may not know that there are special garages that adapt cars for people with disabilities until you meet someone who drives one. A fellow member may tell you about the marvellous Disabled Living Foundation which provides information about all manner of practical aids that could transform your life. (Their address is on p. 225.) Another might have the address of a hotel that is adapted to suit your needs.

Just knowing that there are seventy other people with, for example, motor neurone disease in your county may reduce your sense of loneliness and isolation. It is important to know that you are not suffering alone.

Thinking ahead

Life is going to change—for you, for your family. Stand back, if you can, and find the space to think about yourself, your feelings, your fears. Talk about them, write about them, acknowledge where you are.

Becoming a carer

Becoming a carer is a huge sea change in life. Some people seem to adapt relatively easily to this new and unlooked for role. Others find it much more difficult to come to terms with. Everyone acknowledges that it can be extremely taxing, both physically and emotionally exhausting, sometimes frightening, often depressing. Mixed with all these sad and difficult experiences are equally intense good feelings, feelings of pride, of strength and resilience, of love. Caring for someone you love can be one of the most painful, yet most uplifting, of experiences. Through the pain emerges a real and unshakeable sense of personal worth.

Many of the local and national groups mentioned above will provide great support for carers as well as their loved one. There is also an organization called the Carers National Association (p. 224), which is specifically concerned with the welfare of carers.

Home or hospital

Perhaps you are now ready to think about where you would like to be cared for over the next weeks or months. You may want to consider where you would eventually like to die. To prevent being overwhelmed by the decisions that lie ahead, you need to learn about the options open to you. Understanding how the medical system works may help you to feel more confident about dealing with doctors and nurses and make sure that you get the kind of care and support that you want. Chapter 2 describes the standard of good care that everyone should expect at home. As nearly all terminally ill people spend most of their last year at home, it is essential to understand what medical and social support is available. Britain still has an excellent primary health care system. Everyone has the right to be cared for at home by his or her GP and district nurse, and this care is free at the point of delivery because you have already paid for it in taxes. Many other specialists can also share in your care: hospital and hospice doctors and nurses, social workers, occupational therapists, your priest, your chemist, your home care worker. The list goes on and on. All these people can visit you at home if you need them to do so. Most people who die at home do receive good care. For those whose care does fall short, Chapter 2 ends with a discussion about what you as patient or carer can do to change an unsatisfactory situation.

Most people will spend at least some time in hospital when they are terminally ill, and over fifty per cent of us die in hospital. In what circumstances would a hospital or hospice be a better choice for you? Chapter 3 explores what it can be like to be terminally ill in a hospital or hospice.

As your illness changes, your feelings about being at home, in hospital or in a hospice may also change. It may be unrealistic to say 'Oh, this is how I feel today so I will make a definite decision about A, B or C and then I will stick to it.' For most people it is not like that. Symptoms change, feelings change, life is in flux. Some people need the safety and familiarity of home, the power and control it affords. Others find that they want to be surrounded by experts, or they flourish in the supportive atmosphere of their local hospice or community hospital. It is as well to keep an open mind, for, in order to achieve the best quality of life, you will need to make use of both home and hospital services. The following chapters look at the various options which are open to you and consider what might affect your decisions at different times in your illness.

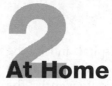

2
At Home

David Williams lived his whole life in the Lake District. When he was sixty-five he developed a cancer of the bladder and was sent from his local hospital to a great specialist centre in Manchester where he received the finest treatment available. He was there for four weeks. His GP visited him when he came home and his first words to her were, 'Oh doctor, thank God I'm home. You won't send me away again will you?' Of course she didn't. Rather than die in the ward of a hospital in Manchester, he was able to live his last months at home surrounded by the lakes and mountains that he had always loved.

Being at home allows patients greater opportunity to determine their own care. It is a way of maintaining control. At home you remain yourself, surrounded by the objects and people that help define you. When profound changes are taking place within your body and your life, the constancy and familiarity of the home environment become particularly important. It is not surprising that given the choice most people prefer to be cared for at home.

At present over half of us die in hospital and about a quarter die at home. A further fourteen per cent die in residential or nursing homes. These stark figures disguise the fact that there is a great deal of movement between home and hospital and in the last year of life patients will spend on average ninety per cent of their time at home. Consequently, the quality of care available at home is very important to nearly all patients.

At the beginning of the twentieth century most people still died in their own homes. By its end well over half of all deaths in the UK took place in hospital, yet another indication of the over-medicalization of life. But people are now beginning to reclaim some of the power that has been appropriated by the medical profession, demanding the right to information and the right to make decisions about their own care. In the book *Living Proof; Courage in the Face of AIDS* by Carolyn Jones, Phyllis Marks says this: 'I feel so old when I think of all the treatments I've had. But I've learned a lot. I've learned how to stand up for myself, how to accept a doctor's information and then choose whether or not I should follow his advice.' The chance to be in your own home strengthens your hand. It helps you to have the courage to choose how you want to be treated, how you want to be cared for.

Another reason for the changes we are seeing is that health care is coming under intense financial scrutiny. Home is cheaper than hospital. In recognition of this fact, and in order to facilitate care at home, the Community Care Act came into force in 1993. Social services now have a vital role to play in maintaining people at home if they want to stay there, as we saw in Chapter 1.

Community medical care

In Britain we have a wonderful system of community medical care for which we are rightly envied. Like most people I tend to take it for granted, but it is quite remarkable. Every patient can choose to be cared for at home and has the right to be attended by highly trained district nurses working alongside general practitioners. Your GP and district nurse cannot turn you down, and actually very few would want to. They value and take great pride in the care they provide for dying patients.

One of the hallmarks of good terminal care is effective symptom control. It is impossible to banish all unpleasant symptoms but a good GP and district nurse team can treat most common symptoms as effectively at home as in hospital. If symptom control proves difficult at home the GP can call on the help of several different specialists, both doctors and nurses. Patients can go to see the specialist in hospital, or the specialist can come to see them at home, which is called a domiciliary visit. General practitioners quite frequently arrange these. Probably the best known of the home care nurse specialists is the Macmillan nurse, who looks after cancer patients. She can give expert advice or she can become involved in the long-term care of a patient at home.

Although most symptoms are amenable to effective treatment at home, some are not. These refractory symptoms are controlled better in hospital than at home, and best of all in a hospice. A good GP will recognize when symptom control is inadequate at home and will arrange for the patient to go into hospital. It may only take a few days to bring a troublesome symptom under control and then the patient can return home again.

The backbone of care for patients at home is provided by district nurses working together with GPs and this chapter starts by considering the kind of medical care you can expect from this team. I look at the role of the home care nurses and also consider the other professionals who may be involved in supporting patients at home. The aim of all these people is to help you and your carer maintain the best possible quality of life while you are at home.

Nearly three-quarters of patients receive good or excellent care at home from their district nurse and GP, but a quarter of patients are less satisfied, and one in ten rate the care they receive as very poor. Sadly, this is particularly the case in inner city areas, where poverty, poor housing and the constant movement of people in and out of an area, with the attendant problems of little family or social support, make the provision of good home care fraught with difficulty. Nevertheless, some of the best care I have seen has been provided in Hackney, a poor inner city borough in London. This chapter will concentrate on the good care you can anticipate, but it will also consider what goes wrong sometimes and what you can do about it.

The key worker

Communication between professionals becomes increasingly important as more people become involved. In hospitals and hospices, palliative care teams hold regular meetings to facilitate communication. In my practice the district nurses meet the GPs over coffee after morning surgery. This allows us to discuss the needs of our terminally ill patients on a daily basis. Particularly when there are complicated problems we will visit the patient together. Any decision making is then shared by the patient, his carers, the district nurse and the GP.

Sometimes patients need support from a large number of professionals. For example I have a patient who is regularly visited by the district nurse, GP, specialist palliative care nurse, hospice chaplain, social worker and dietitian. To keep communication flowing the district nurse arranges what is called a multidisciplinary meeting every two months. As the patient is too unwell to attend her carer comes instead. This helps everyone understand their own role in what I would liken to a complicated jigsaw puzzle of support.

Although it is uncommon for so many people to be involved it is always important that someone co-ordinates things. In this case it is the district nurse. As a patient you can choose who you want to be 'in charge'. That is, who do you really trust to understand how things are for you, and to work with you to get the best possible care available? Usually it is your district nurse or GP, but it could be your social worker or home care specialist nurse. Talk to them, and explain that you would like them to be your 'key worker'. It is important to know that there is one special person who is looking after you and who is taking overall responsibility.

The district nurse

District nurses are often the most important professionals involved in the care of a patient who is at home during his last illness. If you have a first-class district nurse you will be cared for superbly.

District nurses are now known as community nurses. They work in teams and there may be as many as twenty covering a 'patch' or area. In my practice area there are seven nurses in the daytime team and another eleven in the evening and night. In some areas there is no night team and so they are not available after 5 p.m. Very often two nurses from the team work particularly closely with each surgery in the area and they develop a good working relationship based on an understanding of each other's working practices. Of course this relationship also fosters better communication, which is crucial. It also means that although there are many nurses in the team, the patient will receive the majority of their care from only those nurses linked with his GP practice. Obviously this is more comforting than having to get to know everyone.

Who's who in the team?

The first person you will probably meet is the nursing sister. She will be an experienced registered nurse who has undertaken additional specialist qualifications in order to work in the community. Currently district nursing sisters take a one-year BSc Hons in Health and Community Practice at university. More important in my view is that most have a wealth of knowledge and expertise gained from working in the community for many years. The nursing sister will make an initial visit to introduce herself and also to ascertain what help you are going to need at home. Following discussion with both you and your carer she will identify your immediate needs and also try to anticipate what help might be necessary in the longer term. This will all be written into a care plan in which she will also set out exactly what support is going to be arranged. The plan is left at your home so that any doctor or nurse who visits can read it and understand what problems are currently being addressed. Once again it is a way of improving communication. It goes without saying that you can read your own care plan. Perhaps you will have some comments to add; if so tell the nurse who will update it as the situation changes. The plan is then implemented. Usually this involves the nursing sister allocating different areas of nursing care to appropriate members of her team, and at this stage you will probably meet the staff nurses. Again these are registered nurses and many are hugely experienced. I work very closely with our both our nursing sisters and staff nurses and we share a lot of decision making. These decisions can be about all aspects of care—ranging from whether a patient will benefit from referral to a day hospice, to which drug and at what dose to prescribe for a particular symptom. Working closely together in this way helps us both emotionally and intellectually. It certainly enhances the quality of care we are able to provide.

The third group of nurses are the health care assistants, who have taken an NVQ and then received additional training. They provide what is known as personal care and in addition may undertake other tasks such as taking blood or dressing minor wounds.

In the evening and at night when your own district nursing team has gone home there is usually a team of night nurses on call. If you need nursing help during the night, say for example your catheter blocks, the night nursing team will come and look after you. They are not a night sitting service and will leave you once their task is done. This service varies from area to area so ask your district nurse what is available to you. She will advise you how and when to contact them.

What do district nurses do?

In 1991 F. Ross produced this summary of the role of the district nurse, and although it is rather technical I include it because it gives a good indication of how broad the role is (from *Key Issues in District Nursing,* Paper 3, District Nursing Association UK).

- Identification of the physical, emotional and social needs of patients in their own homes as well as the wider needs of the community.
- Planning and provision of episodic and continuing programmes of nursing care particularly for the following groups: the chronic sick, disabled, frail elderly, terminally ill and post-operative patients.
- Mobilizing community resources, both professional and voluntary.
- Ensuring continuity of care between home and hospital in both directions.
- Promotion of health and self-care with individuals and groups.
- Rehabilitation.
- Counselling.

This long and rather daunting list shows that district nurses are expected to care for patients in a holistic way. They are not trained just to do dressings and give injections.

How to contact your district nurse

If you are coming home from hospital having being diagnosed with a terminal illness, the hospital should inform your district nurses who might need to come and remove stitches or re-dress a wound. Even if they have no practical task to perform they will be glad to introduce themselves to you. So it may be that without you doing anything they visit you within a few days of your coming home and offer their help and expertise.

If the diagnosis has been made by your GP, the nurses may be told. This varies from surgery to surgery, but generally the doctors and nurses are in daily communication and often meet after morning surgery to discuss patients. You may feel that you want to keep the news of your illness private, especially if the nurses are part of your community. This is understandable, and it is worth talking to your doctor about whom you want to be told. Obviously nurses are professionals and respect their patients' confidentiality, but nevertheless you can say if you are not ready for them to know.

If you come home and the hospital has not arranged district nursing care, you can ask your GP's surgery to arrange it for you. Usually the receptionist will take a message and pass it on to the nurses, or you can ask your GP. Alternatively you can contact them directly yourself—look them up in the telephone directory under Community Nursing Services.

District nurses value their work with terminally ill patients, and see it as one of their most important roles. Those that I have talked to all emphasize how important it is to meet patients with a terminal illness as early as possible regardless of whether or not there is a physical task for them to perform. They want the opportunity to get to know you and your family.

This again raises the difficult question of when an illness is labelled terminal. If a patient with cancer develops secondaries, in spite of the fact that he may still live for many years, the nurses will be happy to pay a visit and explain what help is available if he needs it in the future. Similarly for someone who converts from HIV positive to AIDS. For other patients, it may be simply that you feel your condition is getting worse and you would like to find out if the district nurses can help.

Once you have met the nurses, you can contact them directly. They will give you their office phone number, and if they are out you can always leave a message for them. The nurses I work with are always happy to give advice over the phone and patients ring them if they are worried and need to talk. A nursing sister in Cambridgeshire described being hailed on the street by the coal man. She was looking after his dying wife and he just needed to talk to her about it. The district nurse is often part of the community and as such is a reassuring and approachable figure who is there for you.

How to get the best out of your district nurse

As with all things in life, some nurses are good and some not so good. On the whole they work as a team because no one nurse is going to be available every single day. This means that you will probably be cared for by several nurses, although you should find that most of the care is given by two or three. There are advantages and disadvantages here—clearly if there is one superb nurse and one less good, it will seem a shame if you don't always have the best. On the other hand, you will not always get the worst.

Different nurses are good at different things. One may be wonderful at identifying problems that can be physically solved, but no use at recognizing that you need to talk about how desperate or terrified you feel. Her colleague may visit the next day and just sit and listen and think about your feelings, but leave without sorting out the constipation you have just developed. We live in the real world with all its imperfections, and recognizing that people have different strengths and weaknesses often helps us to exploit them to our own benefit. So try to make the most of what is on offer. What can each nurse best offer you, with what is she most comfortable, which of your needs can she best meet?

The general practitioner

If you have a really good GP you should get excellent treatment at home during the course of your terminal illness. With luck you already have a doctor who knows you, knows your family, may have helped you in difficult times before. In short, you will have someone that you trust. You may be less lucky, however; perhaps you have recently moved, or more likely if you have been in good health for years, your old doctor has retired and there is a new and unfamiliar face behind the surgery desk.

As your GP is often the person you choose as your 'key worker', the professional who co-ordinates all your other care, you need to establish early on which GP is going to look after you. To do this you need to understand how your particular surgery is organized because there are great differences between one general practice and another.

Which GP will care for me?

Every GP is independently contracted to provide continuing and continuous care for her patients. That means care twenty-four hours a day, 365 days a year, year in, year out. This is fairly easy to understand if you are registered with a single-handed doctor. If you are ill you know whom you are going to see. Most patients are now registered with a group practice and patients can choose with which doctor they make an appointment—that is, to some extent they can choose who looks after them. But many big practices such as my own are now operating a system of 'personal lists'. Although we have 13 500 patients registered at our practice only 1000 are on my personal list because I only work part time. I take full responsibility for their care and think of them as 'my patients'. They are encouraged always to see me rather than one of my partners unless it is urgent. This system allows me to get to know them and vice versa and provides continuity of care. Without continuity it can be very difficult for a doctor to understand the complexity of a case in the ten minutes available for the average consultation. The downside to the system, of course, is that it restricts patient choice.

So your choice of doctor will depend on the way your practice is organized. If you do have a choice then, as with the nurses, see who you feel most comfortable with and try mainly to see that person.

What about home visits?

When you need a home visit it is often less easy to control who comes. You can ask for a particular doctor, and generally she will try to be the one who visits. But it could be her half day, or she may have a meeting, or be on holiday, so over time you are likely to meet several of the GPs in the practice. They will all have different strengths and weaknesses. Make sure you do not end up receiving the majority of your care from someone that you find unsympathetic. If this happens you can ask for help. Tell the doctor herself if you can. Try not to say that you find her difficult, rather say something like 'Although I appreciate all that you are doing, I find that I am very comfortable with Doctor X, and hoped he might be able to visit me more often.' Or talk to the nurses, or to another doctor. It can be very awkward for everyone, but it is very important to you.

What about out of hours calls?

In the last five years there has been a sea change in the way GPs organize their on-call work. Most of them now work together in co-operatives. By pooling resources they cut down night and weekend work while making sure that there is always a doctor available to sick patients. Although this works pretty well for mobile patients with minor illness, it is hard to argue that it is a change that has benefited the terminally ill. Complex problems are much better dealt with by a doctor familiar with the case. GPs have been very worried about this and now have national guidelines to help improve the care in this area. These include the practice of 'flagging up' special patients on the co-operative computer. The flag might give a diagnosis, outline of main treatment and instructions always to visit when asked. Often it will include a note that the patient's own GP would like to be contacted if there is a problem. Some GPs still give their own home phone number to patients who are dying. As my practice is fully computerized we are able to leave a print-out of the recent medical notes with the patient. The more information available to the visiting doctor the better.

A few GPs still do their own on-call work, but most who are not in co-ops use the deputizing service. From the patients' point of view the co-op and deputizing service are very similar—the difference being that one employs fully trained deputizing doctors while the other is staffed by local GPs.

Out of hours calls are beginning to be channelled through the telephone answering service NHS Direct, so you may initially find yourself talking to one of their trained nurses. They will either give you advice or make sure you are put through to the appropriate person such as the co-op or deputizing doctors, the night nurses or the ambulance service.

What will your GP do at first?

Your GP may already be very involved with your care. For patients who have suffered from a chronic illness, this care may have been given over many years. Perhaps your GP has recently diagnosed your illness, or sent you up to the hospital where the diagnosis has been made. In such cases she will know all about you. If a diagnosis is made unexpectedly at the hospital, your GP will have to wait either for a phone call or a letter from the hospital before she fully understands what is going on. This can take a few days.

At this stage, when you have recently been given bad news, you may want to see your GP to talk about how you feel and to discuss what will happen next. If you are well enough, now is the time to visit the surgery to talk about things. Make a long appointment if you can. Feel free to take along a member of your family or a friend. Doctors often see people together. The hospice movement has taught us to think about the carer's needs, as well as those of the patient. After all, you are in this together. The patient faces all the losses associated with a terminal illness, all the fear of the unknown and uncontrollable future. The carer faces the overwhelming loss of a loved one, with all its far-reaching implications. But the carer also faces a desperate challenge, that of coping with both natural distress and the difficulties of caring for a much-loved person. Seeing the doctor together reminds her that you are a team, both having needs that must be recognized.

If you are too ill to go to the surgery ask your GP to visit. She may already have planned to come, but the hospital may not yet have notified her that you are home. It is up to you to contact the surgery and request a visit.

What questions do you have at this time?

By the time you see your GP you may have a long list of questions. It may help to write them down before you see her, which will make sure that you don't forget something that is vital. Patient and carer may have different lists, in which case show them to your GP at the beginning of the consultation. She may say that it will take too long to answer all the questions in one go, and you can plan a further meeting.

Lists are good, but remember you probably don't know all the questions you need answering and surprisingly many of your questions will in the end be answered by you and not by a doctor or nurse. Finding a way of understanding your feelings may be more important to you now than knowing about painkillers or hospital appointments. Sitting down and talking about yourself can sometimes be a very good starting point.

At the beginning of a terminal illness it is often useful for your GP to go over with you what has happened so far, and particularly to find out what you understand about it. If there is a hospital discharge letter it may be helpful to go through it together. Your doctor can explain the diagnosis and talk to you about your future treatment and care. She can give you some idea of what is likely to happen to you in the forthcoming months.

This is a process that many families need to go through again and again. Ask your consultant, ask your GP, ask the nurses. It takes a long time to assimilate all the information that is suddenly being thrown at you. Don't be afraid to repeat yourself.

Further care

Once you have talked to your GP you will have a better idea of how your care is to be organized. Often the hospital will continue to see you. The GP will be someone you can come back to if you need to talk about anything that is confusing or difficult. Your GP should act as your advocate, making sure that you get the best possible treatment available from the hospital service.

Your GP, working with your district nurse, can arrange other professional support for you at home if you need it. Remember, it is your family and your illness and you can decide how much help you want. All decisions should be made with you and not simply made for you.

If getting to the surgery becomes difficult your GP will start to visit you at home. In the latter stages of an illness this can mean weekly visits, and towards the end you will often find the doctor coming in every day.

Unfortunately GPs now do less home visiting than they used to, and in a recent study the most frequent criticism of GPs was reluctance or failure to visit. Visiting is time-consuming. It can take me two hours, including travelling time, to make five visits. In two hours I can see sixteen patients in surgery. But visiting is immensely satisfying, and most GPs enjoy seeing patients in the context of their own homes. Visiting the dying is a central part of the GP's role and no one wants to see that changed.

Symptoms

Tell your GP about any new symptoms you develop. The cause of most symptoms can be satisfactorily diagnosed at the surgery or at home. Sometimes tests are needed. Blood and urine tests can be done at home. Some GPs also have portable ECG (electro-cardiogram) machines to test the heart at home. I personally don't know of anyone with a portable X-ray machine, so for that kind of test you need to go up to the hospital.

Not only can GPs diagnose many things at home, they can also treat most people very effectively. All but the most sophisticated painkilling techniques can be practised at home. It is commonplace for GPs to give morphine. For patients who can no longer swallow, diamorphine can be given under the skin using a small machine called a syringe driver. In a hospital or hospice the treatment is just the same and, indeed, this is the case with most symptoms. Chapter 5 (p. 157) looks at symptom control in more detail.

If your symptoms persist in spite of the best efforts of your GP and district nurse it is very important that you are offered further help. If you have cancer, a home care specialist nurse or hospice doctor may be able to suggest a treatment that makes all the difference. Sometimes it may be necessary to go into hospital. Unfortunately even the most skilled specialists working at the cutting edge of technological medicine cannot manage to banish all symptoms but they can work wonders with some. It is always worth asking them to try.

Emotional support

Patients and carers both need emotional support and this should be part of the overall care provided by the GP. Whereas all doctors can diagnose and treat symptoms, it is not true to say that they will all be able to offer effective emotional support. I think this is a matter of temperament and it is very hard to change doctors who feel uncomfortable dealing with their patients' psychological problems. With training, 'Doctor Brisk' and 'Doctor Grumpy' can develop some of the skills for comforting but such change is neither easy nor common. If your GP cannot respond to your emotional needs, cannot even offer you her sympathy, then make sure you also have support from someone else who can.

The following true stories demonstrate the kind of care a patient can expect to receive from a good GP and district nurse working together with other professionals. They are not unusual or exceptional cases.

Case history

Peter Jenkins was a kind and dignified man who had worked as a crane driver for many years. Both his parents had died of cancer and he had a terror of the disease, which was compounded when his sister-in-law died in great distress from cancer in 1986. A combination of circumstances had conspired against her. She had moved to be with her sisters when she became ill and consequently was away from her own community and her own doctor. There was poor communication between the hospital, her family and the community nurses. But most significantly of all, she had registered with a new GP who did not care. The only home visit she made was to certify the death of her patient.

Several years later Mr Jenkins was diagnosed as having cancer of the stomach. He had an operation which gave him hope of a cure but his wife, Audrey, knew that traces of the tumour remained. A district nurse visited them as soon as they got home and, after talking to them both, left her number and said they should call when they needed her.

Mr Jenkins had four good months and then he began to feel ill. Mrs Jenkins knew his disease was spreading.

She describes the feeling of dread she experienced; not only was she going to lose her beloved husband but she was also petrified at the thought of again caring for a relative who was dying at home. When the GP visited she confronted him with her fears, saying 'What worries me is how he is going to die. As God is my maker, I will not let him suffer.' The GP replied with the question 'Will you give me and my team a chance?' Mrs Jenkins knew that there would be a place for Mr Jenkins in the local hospice should he want it and with this to fall back on she was able to trust the GP. She agreed to give him a chance.

As Mr Jenkins became iller the district nurses began to visit every day. During his last month they came twice a day. They were marvellous. On one occasion Mrs Jenkins told one of the nurses how well she felt she cared for him. 'I like to treat him as if he were my own father,' the nurse replied, 'he is such a dignified man.' Now, two years later, Mrs Jenkins says of this nurse, 'The love in her big, big motherly arms. It was like having a mother look after him.'

He also had regular weekly visits from a Macmillan nurse. She too was wonderful and gave both practical and emotional support. She had time for both Mr and Mrs Jenkins. Mrs Jenkins says, 'There was a gentleness about her and a maturity far above her years. She could calm a tempest. Her presence was so soothing it was unbelievable.'

Not all the professional help was wonderful. Towards the end, Marie Curie nurses were staying three nights a week. One was terrible. The moment she arrived at ten o'clock her first words were 'I've got to leave at 7 a.m. sharp'. Of course, the great majority of the care was given by Mrs Jenkins herself, supported by her family and neighbours. Her sister lifted a great burden by helping with housework and doing all the laundry. A neighbour came in every morning to shave Mr Jenkins.

A brother-in-law sat with him some afternoons to give Mrs Jenkins a break. Being the main carer was so stressful, so demanding and so tiring that as she walked to the hairdresser during one of these brief respites Mrs Jenkins thought 'I'm free, I'm free. Wouldn't it be lovely to run away from all this and never come back.'

Two months before he died Mrs Jenkins told her husband that he was not going to get better, that his cancer was growing again. She didn't want to tell him but all the doctors and nurses urged her to, saying it would be for the best. When she finally did, he cried out 'No, no, no don't tell me, don't take my life away. I've got so much life to live.' Telling eased her burden of secrecy and pretence but she believes he would rather never have known.

At the doctor's regular visits all Mr Jenkins' symptoms were reviewed. Although his pain was completely controlled, nausea remained a problem. Sometimes the doctor would say 'Hospital?' and Mr Jenkins would shake his head. Three weeks before he died Mr Jenkins decided to stop eating. Food made his sickness worse and he hated the indignity of vomiting. From then on he took only iced water. When he could no longer take anything by mouth his drugs were given continuously under the skin using a syringe driver. Then, three nights before he died, he became very agitated and confused. It was ten at night and his wife was alone with him. His GP used the deputizing service at night, but because Mr Jenkins was dying he had given them his home phone number. When Mrs Jenkins phoned he came straight over and was able to settle and calm Mr Jenkins by sitting and soothing him. Before the GP left he gave a small dose of a sedative to help Mr Jenkins sleep through the night.

Mrs Jenkins had a twin sister, Ruthy, who was coming from South Africa to say goodbye and to be with her sister. Mr Jenkins' final goal was to stay alive until she came. When she arrived he was semi-conscious but he seemed to know she was there. His wife held his hand and said to him, 'Well, we done it my darling, didn't we. We reached our goal. My Lord gave me the strength to look after you, and you died as you wanted, you stayed where you wanted and we saw it through.' He squeezed her hand for the last time, a gentle yes in reply.

Mrs Jenkins still comes regularly to the surgery to see her GP. Having known her husband, known how she overcame her fear and with great strength and determination cared for him so well, he is a good person to help support her through her bereavement.

This was a death that was not tidied away as if it were something to be ashamed of. It took its place as it should, as part of the normal and natural life of the community. Friends and family were able to perform really useful caring roles and Mr and Mrs Jenkins were able to enrich the lives of many people by coming through the experience with them.

The story of Mrs Christmas, who was eighty-five and lived alone, is very different.

Case history

Mrs Christmas was a character, very cantankerous, always swearing, cursing her doctors, cursing everyone. She became ill in March and went into hospital where an inoperable lung cancer was diagnosed and treated with palliative radiation. The following week the hospital contacted the district nurses to say that Mrs Christmas was coming home. She was discharging herself against medical advice.

She arrived home at lunch time. The district nurse visited at 2 p.m. 'She was sitting in her armchair, wig askew, with her bags unpacked at her feet where the ambulance men had left them. She couldn't get out of the chair and she was all alone. I thought, how the hell am I going to manage this?'

The nurse went into action and by the following day she had organized meals on wheels, home oxygen had been delivered and set up by the local chemist, and she had arranged urgent assessment visits by the home care organizer and the occupational therapist. Subsequently it was arranged that Mrs Christmas' home care assistant would come in twice a day during the week. At 8 a.m. she would make and feed her breakfast, and at 12 a.m. she would help her to eat her meals on wheels plus do anything else that was necessary. Between times Mrs Christmas would be alone except when the district nurses visited at 8.30 a.m. and 3 p.m. In the evening their night team would settle her down and at 10 p.m. a Marie Curie nurse came and cared for her through the night.

The occupational therapist organized a back rest and cot sides for the bed and with these Mrs Christmas could just about pull herself up to a sitting position. When the district nurse left her each morning she would be propped up in bed with the television on and the telephone and a drink (both of which she was too weak to lift) beside her bed.

Her GP visited regularly. She declined to take the steroids he offered for her breathing but later accepted morphine for her pain.

Mrs Christmas had a family who were able to offer financial support although they did not undertake any of the nursing themselves. One night the Marie Curie nurse was sick and they paid for an agency nurse instead. They also arranged for a private nurse to be with her during the afternoons.

After a week she seemed to lose her old spark, became sad and subdued, stopped swearing or being rude. Gradually she slept more and more of the time, and she died two weeks after coming home. The nursing notes the day before she died say 'All care given. Edith asleep.' The following day she was drowsy and semi-conscious when the district nurse arrived but suddenly she brightened up for a while and took some porridge and a dose of morphine. But before leaving on her rounds the nurse rang the family and the GP to say that Edith's condition had deteriorated. Her daughter-in-law arrived and the GP visited. She was unconscious by now. The doctor left and later the nurse returned to give Mrs Christmas her medication. As she sat on the side of the bed to give it she realized that Mrs Christmas had quietly drawn her last breath and died.

This was not a death that took place in the bosom of loving family, nor was there support from friends or neighbours. But it was very much the death that Edith Christmas wanted. She preferred her own company to that of strangers and she was not afraid to die alone in her own home. The community team, stretched to its limits, was able to offer enough care to make this a comfortable and peaceful death.

Specialists involved in care at home

The strength of the community medical system is that all patients are cared for by district nurses and GPs who are generalists, having a very broad experience of caring for many kinds of patients with all kinds of illness. In an age of increasing specialization, this is to be valued. Yet if difficulties arise where particular skills are needed the GP can call on specialist nurses and doctors. As a GP I often find it useful to ask for this kind of help. Sharing the burden of decision making with someone else, someone who specializes in one field, can be very reassuring to me and very beneficial to my patients.

The home care specialist nurse

Home care specialist nurses are highly trained and experienced nurses who mainly but not exclusively work with cancer patients. They are often known by the more familiar name of Macmillan nurses, though there are other such nurses who may take their name from the charities that fund them. In hospital they are called palliative care nurses and they work as part of a hospice or hospital palliative care team that specializes in the care of dying patients. They can also work independently. These nurses bring the special skills of the hospice into the community and are a third and very important group of professionals who care for patients in their own homes.

Most GPs feel that their dying patients should all have equal access to home care specialist nurses and hospice care. One GP I know described the specialist cancer and palliative care services as 'diseasist' and I go along with that. If you are one of the majority of patients who are dying of something other than cancer you probably will not have access to a specialist nurse. Ask your GP and your hospital consultant if a specialist nurse is available to you. If there is not, rest assured that with a good GP and district nurse your care will be equally as good.

Not all cancer patients have access to the service either. In some rural areas there is still no access to domiciliary palliative care services.

In the UK over 120 000 patients a year are seen at home by palliative care nurses and this is well over half of all patients dying of cancer. Patients are under their care at home for an average three to four months.

Although doctors have legitimate grumbles about who has access to home care nursing, they can only acknowledge the excellence of the care which is provided. Home care nurses look after fewer patients than district nurses and this gives them more time to spend with each one. It is this wonderful gift of time that enables them to provide such good total care. They have time to sit and listen, and they are trained to hear what you are saying (listening for the real meaning of a patient's words is so important). Offering extra emotional and psychological support to patient and carers is central to their role, something for which they are very highly valued. Home care nurses bring to this the hospice ideals of openness and respect for the patient's autonomy. Their primary concern is for quality of life, helping their patients to live the life that is left to the full.

They are also experts at symptom control, and will be up to date with all the latest advances in treatment. No symptom is too trivial.

All home care specialist nurses, whether working alone or as part of a team, will have regular contact with a doctor, either the GP or a hospital doctor who specializes in care of the dying. She can discuss any difficult problems with them before recommending treatment. For those nurses who work as part of a hospice team regular contact with the specialist allows problems to be remedied speedily—they have a fast track to the experts. They also have the added advantage of meeting regularly with the social or welfare worker and others who may be helpful to you. When contemplating admission to a hospice, either as a day patient or an inpatient, the specialist nurse helps facilitate arrangements and, most importantly, the patient has the additional comfort of seeing a familiar face on the wards.

How do you feel about accepting a home care specialist nurse?

Everyone knows that Macmillan nurses care for the dying. Although some patients readily and gratefully accept the suggestion that they be visited by a home care specialist nurse, others do not. Perhaps it feels like giving up the fight for life and often that is the last thing you want to do. You might think 'OK, I know that I've got cancer, I've come to terms with that. But I'm not going to die yet, I'm not even going to think about it.' Determination to live and to fight the disease are feelings that need supporting and encouraging. But if you have symptoms that are not controlled your fighting spirit will be weakened. Similarly if you sense that you are only just keeping the lid on your anxiety, pushing your fear deep down inside, most of your energy is being used up and wasted fighting to keep control.

In my experience home care nurses are empathic rather than just sympathetic. Imagine what a relief it might be to meet someone who really cares about how you are feeling, who has time for you, who wants to understand. Imagine having someone for whom no worry or symptom seems too trivial and who is skilled at treatment. Imagine being cared for by someone who respects your autonomy, and thinks about your welfare in the context of your whole family, who cares about your carers. It may be scary to admit that you are ready to accept their support but your courage may be richly rewarded.

How to contact them

You can be referred by your GP, district nurse, hospital doctor, or you can refer yourself. The home care specialist nurse always checks with your GP before she becomes involved so that there is no confusion about who is doing what. It is a very rare GP who does not welcome her involvement.

Commonly your GP or district nurse refers you if they are having a problem with symptom control. They should always discuss the referral with you first. The specialist nurse then works alongside the GP and district nurse. She may suggest some new treatment, or help rationalize the current regime. Your GP will then prescribe what is needed, and between them the team will monitor the troublesome symptoms until they are settled. This may mean that at times the specialist nurse will come in every day, or even more frequently. Your district nurse will usually continue to provide regular care, as will your GP. Unfortunately the specialist nurses do not do much 'hands on' nursing so they may ask your district nurse to administer some treatments like enemas or catheterization.

It is essential that you understand who is doing what. Keep in mind the idea of a key worker so that you have one person you trust to oversee your care. Even though a specialist nurse is helping, you may still feel that your district nurse or GP is that key person. On the other hand, if you need continuing intensive care from the specialist nurse she may become the key worker for you. As ever, choose the person in whom you feel most confidence and find most comfortable to be with.

A specialist nurse is often asked to get involved when your GP and district nurses are unable to give enough time to the emotional needs of you or your carer. Larger palliative care teams often have a bereavement support worker and the specialist nurse may continue to visit the bereaved carer. We know that support for the bereaved is woefully inadequate and the palliative care services rightly give it very high priority.

Hospice at home

Hospice at home is another service that is worth exploring as it becomes increasingly available across the UK where there are now 78 of them. Most but not all are run from the local hospice. I have recently used the service very successfully with one patient. As she drew near the end her nursing needs became too great for her family to manage even with full district and palliative care specialist nurse support. Rather than send her into the local hospital or hospice we called in the hospice at home service. Three nurses came and provided round-the-clock nursing care at home for the last few days of my patient's life. When I visited I felt the atmosphere in the house had become calm and quiet and it was noticeable that although the family continued to look after their loved one the burden of full responsibility had been lifted from their shoulders. It was a very peaceful death.

Different areas provide different kinds of hospices at home. These vary from highly organized rapid response teams who will provide complicated medical care at home such as blood transfusions, to others who provide less intense ongoing nursing and social support such as regular respite care. To find out what, if anything, is available in your area ask your district nurse or contact your local hospice. This is another excellent service we need to develop so that it can be available to everyone who needs it.

Other specialist nurses

There are specialist nurses for all sorts of other diseases: children with cystic fibrosis or heart disease, for example; patients with Parkinson's or motor neuron disease. Ask your hospital specialist if there is a nurse in your area for patients with your disease.

Another group of specialist nurses are those who are expert at particular kinds of symptom control, such as incontinence nurse specialists and stoma care specialists. Your district nurse will put you in contact with them if necessary. Access to a specialist nurse is limited, unfortunately, and in many areas and for many diseases there will be no specialist nurse available.

Night nurses are a most valuable resource, arranged for you by your district nurse. They will look after a patient through the night in order to allow the carer to sleep undisturbed and they provide full nursing care. Some are highly trained, others are not. Usually they are charitably funded, the Marie Curie Foundation provides their own nurses, for example.

Because a night nurse is there through the long night hours she can often be someone in whom patients and carers confide, a bit like a stranger on a train to whom you tell your most intimate secrets. They can also play an important role in symptom control as they have the opportunity to monitor the patient's condition undisturbed over several hours.

Night nurses appreciate being looked after a little themselves. They need a comfortable chair with a reading light and somewhere to make a cup of tea. The night is a long time to keep awake.

Once again, however, this wonderful service is not available to everyone. Marie Curie nurses work exclusively with cancer patients and are in short supply. On average a patient dying at home from cancer will receive only four sessions of care in total from Marie Curie nurses and, if anything, the service is getting worse rather than better. Those with other diseases are unlikely to find any overnight nurse available on the NHS. Ask your district nurse if there is any help in your area. The absence of a comprehensive night sitting service is a woeful inadequacy in the care provided to the chronic sick and terminally ill in Britain.

Specialist doctors

Hospice doctors or palliative care specialists can be invited by the GP to make a home visit. Sometimes they come in an advisory role, to help with difficult symptoms. Hospice doctors may want to meet patients and carers in the context of their home before they are admitted to a hospice. They are very useful to me as a GP and I often telephone them for advice.

It is less common to ask for a domiciliary visit from a hospital consultant but at times it can be useful. A psychiatrist can visit if a patient becomes very depressed or distressed, a physician if there is a difficult medical problem. A geriatrician often makes home visits to elderly patients. Because of their special knowledge of the problems associated with old age, they often help the GP and district nurse resolve difficulties at home without the patient being admitted to hospital.

Other sources of support

The list of professionals and others who may provide support could go on and on. Physiotherapists, speech therapists, complementary therapists, etc. may all be involved in supporting patients at home during a terminal illness, although those detailed below are the people with whom you are most likely to come into contact. They can be accessed through social services, a hospital social worker or the GP/district nurse team.

Social worker

Many patients who suffer from a chronic illness will already have a social worker. Others may have been put in touch with one at the hospital. Most patients still never see a social worker as part of the care they receive at home, although nearly everyone would benefit from their help. They will arrange a co-ordinated assessment of your needs and for the provision of services, as outlined in Chapter 1. Just as important is their role in giving psychological and emotional support, and hospital social workers particularly see this as an integral part of their job.

Occupational therapist

Although an occupational therapist is unlikely to be involved on a day-to-day basis, a home visit can be of immense benefit. He or she assesses what aids will help you to continue to function independently as your disease progresses. They can provide all sorts of equipment, from expensive items such as stair lifts and shower fittings down to specially adapted cutlery and drinking straws.

Home care worker

With a growing population of elderly patients, many of whom live alone, a home care assistant can be a lifeline. For some they clean and tidy, for others they do the shopping or the laundry. Some will help get you up, dressed and washed. They also provide company and contact with the world outside the front door, and generally keep an eye on things.

There are not enough home care assistants, and therefore they are allocated according to need, which often means that the elderly who live alone are prioritized.

Minister of the church

If you have a religious faith you may already be supported by your minister. If not you can always contact one for the first time. In hospital there are usually priests of many faiths available who can talk with you about spiritual matters. But equally you may wish to discuss other business, such as the arrangements for your funeral. Priests who are comfortable working with dying people (by no means all) have broad skills; they can listen and counsel, they can often arrange social support, church visitors and sitters, they even learn a lot about good medical care although they would probably never claim this as part of their job. One experienced vicar told me that he had learnt how important it was to treat constipation in the terminally ill. He knew that only when this troublesome symptom had been treated would a person be ready to talk about spiritual matters.

Chemist

Your chemist or pharmacist can be someone who simply dispenses your prescription or he can be another source of valuable support. Ideally you need to get to know your pharmacist and his staff.

Your pharmacist will understand that you need medicine fairly urgently when you are terminally ill, that it is no good saying, 'We will have that in for you in three days' time' because you cannot wait that long. Neither is it helpful to hear, 'That will be ready for collection at 4 p.m.' when it is 10 a.m. and this is your only chance of getting out of the house for the day. One of the ways pharmacists look after their clients is to deliver drugs to their home, and sometimes they also pick up your prescriptions from the surgery.

Pharmacists are great experts on drugs, how they interact and possible side effects. You can always ask them if you have a query about your drugs. Patients who are elderly or confused may be supplied with special tablet dispensers called dosset boxes by a thoughtful pharmacist.

So choose your pharmacist with care, explain your situation and ask what he or she can do to help you.

Special association volunteers

Age Concern volunteers, Church Council volunteers, Hospice volunteers, AIDS 'buddies': there is a long list of potential helpers that are worth investigating because the statutory services fall very short in their ability to provide adequate support services. Volunteer help can range from the purely practical like a lift to the hospital or shops, to a deeper and more supportive friendship.

What can go wrong

Sadly some people are not well cared for at home when they are dying. There are a number of reasons for this and I will list those that are most common.

Poor communication

One prerequisite for good care is good communication—between patient, carer, GP, district nurse, specialist nurses, hospital specialist, junior doctors, ward staff. It is quite a tall order to maintain good channels of communication with such a large and geographically spaced group. I can think with embarrassment of many of my consultations that have taken place without all the relevant medical information available. Hospitals are no better. Notification of an important appointment arrives too late for you to attend. Or you are sent home from hospital expecting full nursing services to have been arranged and nobody comes. Often when you feel let down like this the fault lies not with the individuals concerned but with the administration of the whole complex system. This is no excuse, however, and for you as a patient each failure seems like a personal blow. You think 'they have lost my notes, they don't really care about me'; 'the district nurses never bothered to visit when the hospital had made arrangements, so clearly they don't care how I am'. On the whole the professionals themselves do care, but the 'system' makes them appear not to.

Lines of communication are particularly easily broken when a patient moves, and this is a very common problem. It is what happened to Mrs Jenkins' sister (see p. 46). Not so long ago families used to live for generation after generation in the same place. Nowadays society is more mobile; children move for work or education, retirement often gives people the opportunity to move to the country, to the sea, or even abroad. But family ties remain strong, and in times of illness, particularly a terminal illness, family members want to look after each other. Often the only way of doing this is to move the patient to the carer. Consequently, in general practice doctors are used to looking after ill patients who are in the area *because* they are ill. It is not ideal for the patient who probably has a doctor at home he has known and trusted for years, and it is not ideal for the doctor or nurse who has to get to know the patient and his illness from scratch. As a compromise, however, it works very well provided communication is good. Every patient has the right to register with a local doctor when away from home and in need of medical care. If you have moved to be near your family it is usual to sign on with their doctor as a temporary resident.

Personally I appreciate it if a carer comes to see me before the patient arrives. We can discuss what help will be needed and, if necessary, I can speak to the patient's own GP or the hospital so that I understand the case. Very often a patient arrives to stay with relatives on a Friday afternoon and temporary support arrangements have to be made for the weekend when services are at their scarcest. It is much less fraught if everything has been planned in advance.

Personality clashes

You feel comfortable with some doctors and nurses, with others you do not. This is not necessarily a reflection of how 'good' they are at their work, or of how sympathetic and kind they are. As with all relationships, it is often difficult to identify exactly why the chemistry works. If the chemistry is badly wrong you will need to talk to another nurse or your GP about the problem, and this takes a certain degree of courage. In general practice it is understood that different doctors suit different patients and the same is true of nurses. An experienced health professional will recognize that the quality of relationship with the patient will affect the quality of care he or she is able to provide. So if you are unhappy with a particular doctor or nurse it is well worth acknowledging this and trying to do something about it.

The doctor or nurse who lets you down

What if you feel let down by your doctor or nurse, and this undermines the trust you have placed in them? This can happen, and it is a shame because although professionals often fail you in some ways it is not always because they do not care. The task of looking after a dying patient stretches even the best doctors and nurses and, sadly, in spite of good intentions things go wrong. Common examples are that your doctor gives you bad news badly; or the GP you like and trust fails to diagnose a chest infection which results in a hospital admission. My heart sinks when this happens to me, not least because I know some junior doctor will probably make a disparaging remark, undermining my whole credibility as a competent doctor. Perhaps your nurse forgets to visit, or is grumpy when you ask her to come. Sometimes she is on holiday or ill when you most need her, and this makes you understandably angry with her. The important thing is to differentiate those who are doing their best but who sometimes let you down from those who really do not care.

The uncaring doctor

Why some doctors do not care about their dying patients is a big and interesting subject. However, for the patient registered with such a doctor there is nothing interesting about it, it is just an unmitigated disaster. What are you going to do? With group practices you are on fairly safe ground as generally one of the other partners will be providing good terminal care. Ask your district nurse to tell you who will look after you best, and fight to get the doctor you want.

If you have a good district nurse she will make sure that you are well cared for. If you have little faith in either your GP or district nurse see if you can involve a home care specialist nurse.

A really poor and uncaring doctor is luckily a rare thing, but they do exist. If you are registered with a single-handed practitioner and are unable to mobilize any alternative support, as a last resort you may have to change doctors.

Case history

Louise Cornford had recently moved house to be near her daughter, when she suddenly developed lumps behind her neck and became weak and ill. She had recently registered with a local doctor so she rang and asked for a visit. The doctor said she was busy and would come when she could. Two days later no visit had been made and by then the woman was in pain. Her son telephoned the GP and demanded that she visit. 'Well is it a matter of life and death?' she said, still unwilling to come. 'No,' he replied 'it's a matter of quality of dying' and put down the phone. He rang his sister's GP who visited straight away, and agreed without hesitation to look after her.

The GP who will not ask for help

The other, more difficult scenario is the GP who likes to be in control of all aspects of her patient's care. Although she is not achieving good symptom control or providing emotional support she does not want anyone else to 'interfere' and will not readily involve the district nurse. She certainly will not welcome the home care specialist nurse.

If your doctor clearly does not give a damn it seems to me the choice of action is relatively simple—change doctor. With a GP who cannot provide you with good care but will not ask for help, it is much more difficult. If your GP has always looked after you well in the past the notion of leaving her care is almost unthinkable. It is like denying the trust that you and your family have rightly put in her for years. But if, for example, she fails to control your pain, refuses to hear your distress, prevents you from getting the help you need from other professionals, then perhaps you will have no option. It is a decision that should only be taken after very serious consideration.

How to change doctor

In recent years it has been made much easier for patients to change their GP. Gone are the days when you had to get signed off by your old doctor before you could register with a new one. These days you simply go to the new surgery and ask to be taken on. You don't even have to produce your old medical card, although it helps if you can. A practice does have the right to refuse to register any new patient and by far the commonest reason for refusal is that you do not live near enough to the surgery. Patients who move locally will usually be kept on by their own GP even though they live some distance away, but new patients must live within a certain demarcated area. If you do decide to change doctor, try asking the district nurses whom they would recommend.

Summary

Studies have shown that seventy per cent of patients receive good or excellent care from their district nurse and GP. Away from the inner cities this figure is even higher. I hope that those who are not satisfied with the care they receive will be able to use the information in this chapter to change things for the better.

At home you remain yourself, you are the king in your castle and your GP and district nurses will provide you with continuing care, and you should have access to all kinds of specialist help if you need it. This gives you power and control. One carer said to me, 'I didn't want someone to take over, but to come and share the care', and this partnership of equals is really only possible when you are at home.

3
Hospital, Hospice or Home?

You may have a strong feeling from the outset about where you would like to be cared for, particularly towards the end. Or you may never have thought about it, or realized that you might have a choice. At the beginning of a terminal illness most patients say that they would prefer to die at home rather than in hospital. Towards the end of their illness about half say hospital or hospice. So some patients change their minds, usually in the direction of hospital and hospice. Being allowed to change your mind is very important.

At the other end of life there is a good example of how rigid expectations can be detrimental. Having a baby at home is for some women a choice that they desperately want to make, and a home birth is undoubtedly an experience to be treasured. But we are dealing with the raw force of nature, here, which refuses always to be controlled. Sometimes a couple who have planned and often fought with their doctors and midwives for the right to have a home birth, are foiled by nature herself. The baby will not come, mother and child are in danger and need medical help that is only available in hospital. So in they go, and in due course the baby is safely delivered. Surely this is a moment to celebrate, to feel proud of—the fact of the new life is so momentous that the place of birth is of secondary importance. That is not to say that it is unimportant, but it should not stand in the parents' way and spoil their celebration. Yet sometimes I have seen it do just that. The couple wanted a home birth so badly that they could take little pleasure in the hospital delivery. Home means being yourself, staying in control, and going into hospital feels like losing control at a frightening and painful time. But with both birth and death we are unable to be in total control. Before you settle too strongly on the place in which you wish to die, remember that circumstances change and your feelings may change. You cannot necessarily remain in total control because you are dealing with nature and she is in fighting mood. Planning ahead a little helps you identify your options and only by understanding the alternatives can you decide what will be best for both you and your carers.

Hospital care

Case history

When I was a junior doctor working all the hours that God gave me on a busy medical ward, an octogenarian was admitted one night following a dense stroke. He was unconscious. I examined him, passed a catheter into his bladder to save him lying in a wet bed and then it was a matter of waiting to see what was going to happen. Initially he was admitted to the open ward, but after a short time, when it became apparent that he has unlikely to survive for long, sister moved him into a side room and telephoned his wife, who came straight up to the hospital. She was a little bird-like figure also in her eighties to judge from her appearance. Her husband lived for two more days and most of this time she sat by his bed holding his hand. On the third day as I was passing the room she appeared in the corridor and said that he had stopped breathing. I went in to find that indeed he had died, apparently peacefully, having never regained consciousness. She was not surprised when I returned to confirm what she already knew, that her husband was dead. I asked if she would like to go in to see him and when she looked unsure I said 'Would you like me to go in with you?' So we went in together. I stood just inside the door. She went around the bed and after regarding her husband for a few seconds leant over and kissed him on the lips. She said 'Thank you for fifty wonderful years, my darling.' Tears were welling in my eyes as we left the room and I expect they were in hers too although it is so long ago that I can't remember now.

This death was apparently peaceful and easy for the patient although we can never really know what an unconscious mind may be experiencing. For his wife it was a good death. She was able to be with her husband to the end but was relieved of the burden of nursing him. In an unconscious patient this burden is considerable, turning the patient every three hours, bathing him, changing his bed daily. She was able to be alone with him while he was alive but after his death preferred to have me with her, as a result of which I had the great privilege of witnessing her final goodbye.

For many people it is better to die in a hospital or hospice than at home. Trying to decide which is going to be best for you or your loved one is extremely difficult as so many unpredictable factors will affect your experience. But there are also many factors that we can predict, and considering the various aspects may help you make a balanced judgment about where you would like to be.

I have started this chapter by illustrating a 'good death' in hospital because, after all, that is what this book is about. Why was this a good death? Well, firstly the sister was skilful, identifying early that her patient was dying, calling his wife immediately so that she could be with him for what little time they had left and, luxury of luxuries, giving them a side room to protect them from the bustle of normal ward life. (They were lucky, often there is no side room available.) There was no restriction on visiting so the patient's wife could stay as long as she wanted. To give my youthful self credit, I too was sensitive, feeling her apprehension and yet understanding that to say farewell is so important.

Of course the nature of his illness was also an important factor. A stroke of this sort is not amenable to heroic medical intervention and so the patient's death was untroubled by drips, drugs or surgery. It was therefore peaceful.

Many carers are over the age of sixty-five, and an increasing number are over eighty. As my patients often say 'Old age never comes alone', by which they mean that chronic illness is their sad companion. When you are eighty it is hard enough to care for your sick spouse, but how much harder when you are eighty with arthritis in the hands and knees, angina and shortness of breath. Yet such people do sometimes manage to remain the prime carer at home, often taking the attitude 'I've cooked and looked after him for fifty years and I'm not going to stop now'. As a society we can acknowledge their strength and their remarkable determination, but we should also make sure that they do this by choice and not because there is no caring and dignified alternative.

The little bird-like woman went home to live alone, and thus became one of the growing population who often come into hospital to die—elderly single people. Recently I cared for just such a woman who had nursed her husband through his terminal illness at home two years previously. Now she too was dying of a cancer of the lining of the lungs called mesothelioma.

Case history

Mrs O'Neil had known about her diagnosis and prognosis almost since her husband's death, and she also understood the misfortune of her situation. Mesothelioma is a tumour caused by exposure to blue asbestos and many years before she had been unknowingly exposed by washing her husband's work shirts. She must have breathed in small fibres as she shook the shirts out and now years later they were killing her. Mesothelioma is an industrial disease and throughout the last year of her life she was pursuing a claim against the company that had employed her husband and exposed them both to asbestos. In this she was supported by her hospital consultant who had written several long and complicated reports on her behalf. Sadly she died before the case was settled.

Mrs O'Neil was very clear that she wanted to die in hospital. She liked and trusted her consultant, and knew the ward staff well from frequent admissions in the past. In the last six months of her life fluid built up around the tumour making her compromised breathing even worse. Whenever it got too difficult she asked to be sent into the ward where they would draw off the fluid. These admissions lasted three or four days and gave her relief from her symptoms; they also gave her a rest from looking after herself and a change of scene. Finally the sad day came when no more fluid could be drawn off, only the growing tumour was left. Mrs O'Neil came home for the last time. She had a birthday tea with her family and the district nurses. A few days later her breathing became worse and she asked to go back to hospital. There she died within a week, not alone, not among strangers, but in the care of the medical staff that she had grown fond of and who had grown fond of her. It was as she wanted it.

Why hospital?

Why did Mrs O'Neil choose to die in hospital? It is worth looking at her reasons in more detail and then considering some factors that can play a part in other cases.

Dying alone

Mrs O'Neil did not want to die alone at home. Over thirty per cent of people in Britain live alone during the last year of their lives. Younger people who live alone usually have friends and family to surround and care for them. But the tragedy for our old people is that many outlive their friends and family, and are left quite alone and isolated. Although a few choose to maintain their independence to the end, most wearily accept the need to go into either a hospital or nursing home. Yet for socially isolated people the hospital ward can seem like a large family. One old lady I visited after she had been in hospital for treatment said 'Oh, it was lovely in there. I was the oldest patient on the ward and they made a tremendous fuss of me. They even made me a birthday cake for my eighty-first birthday and everyone sang happy birthday.'

Poor symptom control

Poor symptom control is one of the main reasons that patients need to go into hospital. For many a short stay is all that is required and once control has been achieved they can go home. Increasing weakness and shortness of breath, for example, may be due to anaemia. After a day in hospital and a blood transfusion the symptoms will be better. This treatment can be given at home but most GPs prefer to admit patients to hospital for such procedures.

Pain control is, of course, another reason for hospitalization. There is good evidence that symptom control is better in hospital than at home and it is at its best in the hospices. Again, within a few days, troublesome pain may be controlled and the patient can return home. For some people, however, long admissions are needed.

Emergency admissions

Quite often patients are rushed into hospital when an unanticipated emergency arises or, as in the following case, where the community services fail to respond adequately.

Case history

Anne Reed had multiple sclerosis for fifty years. Nine months before she died she had a stroke and although she regained consciousness she never spoke again. One evening Mr Reed noticed that his wife was groaning and shaking. He watched for a while hoping that this would cease but it gradually became worse. He called the surgery but it was shut and he was put through to the deputizing service. They said a doctor would come. After two hours no doctor had arrived and so in desperation he called an ambulance. It took both of them straight to hospital. Anne was put in a cubicle and Mr Reed sat outside. After half an hour the nurse came out and said that Anne had died. Mr Reed was in shock and he still cannot remember how he said goodbye to his wife, whether he kissed her or not.

Anne died of a stroke and there was no indication even a few hours earlier that death was imminent. Mr Reed had cared for her devotedly for many, many years. The manner of her death left him feeling confused: 'Sometimes I wonder if I should have called an ambulance earlier. Sometimes I regret not seeing her in the chapel of rest because the last time I saw her she was very distressed.' After all those years of care it was a very hard way for him to lose her.

Being a burden to your carers

Mrs O'Neil did not want to die alone but in her case matters were slightly more complicated than that. She had a loving son who lived close by with his family and throughout her illness he expressed his willingness to look after her. But she chose not to accept this offer, I believe, because she did not want to be a burden on anyone. Some people feel very strongly that they do not want their family or friends to have to look after them, and I expect that these are often people who have themselves been burdened with the care of a loved one in the past. And indeed it may be physically impossible for one family to nurse a patient at home.

Shedding the burden of responsibility

The responsibility faced by both patient and carers at home can be very great, and reducing it may take an enormous strain off family relationships which consequently improve. This can be a very important reason for opting for hospital over home care.

The presence of trained staff and modern technology are very reassuring for some patients. At home they feel scared, but in hospital they are much calmer, much happier. When sent home for a while they are reassured by knowing that the ward is there waiting any time they want to go back in.

It is well recognized that the feelings of carers are as important as those of the patient when it comes to choosing the place of care, and sometimes they find it is a great relief to be able to shed some of the responsibility of managing at home. This is particularly true for those carers who become exhausted, anxious and miserable. Sharing the physical and organizational load with the ward staff allows them to concentrate on sharing time with the patient, being there for them emotionally, enjoying each other without always having jobs to do, meals to cook, visitors to attend to.

When a patient dies at home there will inevitably be a room and a bed in which they died. For a few people this is very distressing. They find it a constant reminder of their loss. It can be another reason for choosing hospital rather than home.

Improving carer/patient relationships

Going into hospital can improve the relationship between patient and carer in another way. With the onset of illness, previously independent people can find they are suddenly thrown together for twenty-four hours a day. It seems ungracious to complain of this when you know that your time together is finite. People feel they should treasure every minute. But constant proximity may be unnatural and some relationships suffer greatly. Better to have several good hours together than twenty-four tense and miserable ones.

Which hospital?

You may already know that you want to be in hospital, but even if you feel fairly strongly that home rather than hospital is the place for you it is worth asking some of the following questions.

If you do need to go into hospital for some of your terminal care, which hospital are you likely to go to, and what will it have to offer you as a patient? Have you any choice in the matter? Do you know what alternatives there might be and how do you go about finding out? Finally, what are the logistics of moving between home, hospital or hospice?

Most patients choose to go to the local community hospital or to their district general hospital. But some will be referred to specialist centres for treatment and will make their main relationships with the staff there. An increasing number of elderly people are in residential or nursing homes. Other people may choose referral to a local hospice or a private hospital. The philosophy behind hospice care used to be (and often still is) very different from the approach found on most general wards. However, many hospitals now have specialist palliative care teams who help make sure that dying patients are well looked after. They do this both by educating other members of staff and also by sharing the care of patients who need their help. The teams vary from hospital to hospital but all have one or more specialist nurse, often a palliative care consultant with a team of junior doctors, and sometimes a social worker, occupational therapist, psychologist and chaplain.

If you are in hospital your consultant can refer you to this team for all kinds of reasons such as better symptom control, emotional, spiritual or psychological support, or help in planning your discharge home. It is a team that works alongside your own consultant and ward nurses but does not take over from them completely.

District general hospitals

Most patients are cared for in their local district general hospital, and if your consultant admits you to hospital this is where you will probably go. Most terminally ill patients die in their local district general hospital except in areas served by a community hospital.

Specialist centres

Although the district general hospitals can provide a very high standard of care sometimes more specialization is needed. For example, many cancer patients will be referred on to hospitals that provide joint clinics run by oncologists, radiotherapists and surgeons or physicians. Patients with neurological, liver or renal diseases may have been under the care of a specialist hospital for years. Many AIDS patients travel great distances to specialist centers. When or if active treatment finishes, patients may have the choice of staying under their specialist hospital when they become terminally ill, or of returning to their local hospital.

All specialist centres look after far more patients than they have beds for. When treatment is finished, most patients return to their local hospital for the continuing care which can be provided there just as well, if not better, than in the specialist centre.

Community hospitals

Community hospitals used to be called cottage hospitals. Currently there are over 400 community hospitals in the UK serving twenty per cent of the population. They are mainly found outside the large urban conurbations.

A community hospital is always small—less than 100 beds. GPs look after their own patients in these beds. Consultants sometimes admit patients too. In many ways they are old-fashioned institutions that have weathered years in the wilderness while society worshipped exclusively at the shrine of high-tech medicine. But they survived essentially because they have always been highly valued by the communities they serve. Suddenly the secret of their success is out and they are coming back into fashion.

Community hospitals play a major role in the care offered to dying patients. In areas served by a community hospital, nearly two in five patients with cancer die there. The same is probably true for patients with other terminal diseases. Far fewer patients die in district general and specialist hospitals, and even fewer die at home. Often terminally ill patients who refuse to go into their local general hospital will happily go to their community one. It is local and therefore familiar. The staff are local too. You do not have to get to know a new doctor—your GP looks after you. Patients can go in for treatment that might be difficult at home. You may need a blood transfusion, treatment for breathlessness or intravenous drug therapy. You may need intensive rehabilitation after a stroke. Nursing care is provided by trained nurses and many patients are admitted for this alone. You may need respite care either on a regular basis or as a one-off.

Because they are small and because they are local, community hospitals usually have a homely atmosphere. Many have specially allocated side rooms which are made particularly comfortable for patients who are dying.

The best recommendation will come to you by word of mouth from your local community. If you want more information about the quality of care they provide to patients who are dying you could ask some of the following questions. Does the hospital have a private interview room? What about overnight accommodation for relatives? Do terminally ill patients have the use of special beds or Pegasus mattresses, for example? Have any nurses on the staff completed their ENB 931 continuing care course which gives them special training in the care of terminally ill patients? Positive answers to these questions suggest that good terminal care is one of their priorities.

Private hospitals

You may choose a private hospital, of which there are an increasing number. These are very variable both in the standard of care provided and in cost, so it is worth thinking carefully about which one you choose. Ask your GP and anyone else who may know about the hospital. Ask your consultant about how she cares for her terminally ill patients. If she denies that the question is appropriate in your case because you are not terminally ill, ask again; how would she look after you if you were? Perhaps you could visit and ask the sister in charge how they approach the care of their terminally ill patients. Have any nurses taken the ENB 931 continuing care course? You may get wonderful care but be careful and make sure that you are not paying for a private room and good food at the expense of really good symptom control and attention to all your emotional and spiritual needs.

Residential and nursing homes

As our population ages, more and more people are spending their last days in care homes. Currently this is where twelve to fifteen per cent of us die. Some are owned and run by the local authority but an increasing number are private homes which are run as profit-making organizations. In the private sector, standards of accommodation may be determined by a resident's ability to pay. So, perhaps, may the standard of care received.

Both residential and nursing homes provide care 'until death'. Those that are well and kindly run can become a real home to residents who for one reason for another are incapable of living independently. Unfortunately others resemble the worst of our old-fashioned institutions with no heed paid to the feelings or rights of the clients, and a grim 'them and us' attitude pervasive among the predominantly untrained staff.

Care homes all have to be registered and are subjected to regular inspection. Residential homes are registered with the local authority and provide 'personal care' for people who are relatively independent. Nursing homes are registered with the health authority and because they provide 'nursing care' for a more dependent group of residents they must have a trained nurse on duty at all times. Some homes have dual registration and are often divided into two distinct halves which are staffed separately.

Residents in a residential home who become ill will receive medical care from their GP and local district nurses in much the same way as they would at home. Clearly the staff of the home will be required to look after them as well. National guidelines state that 'the care provided is limited to that appropriate to a residential setting and is broadly equivalent to what might be provided by a competent and caring relative'. Asking how much care a competent and caring relative can provide is like asking how long is a piece of string—it is very imprecise but does give both residents and staff the option of receiving or providing terminal care in the residential home. This is very important for those who have made it their only home. Sometimes a resident's condition cannot be adequately treated under these circumstances and it may be better and kinder to transfer them to a nursing home or hospital.

In all nursing homes terminal care will be provided by the staff of the home supported by the GP. Home care nurse specialists may also visit patients in both residential and nursing homes. In some parts of the country where there is no hospice or community hospital, GPs may admit patients to a local nursing home specifically for terminal care.

The standard of terminal care is extremely variable in both residential and nursing homes. In the worst cases the dying person is isolated, seemingly hidden away with no attempt made to acknowledge his or her feelings or those of other residents. Symptom control will largely depend on the level of interest and skill of the sister in charge and on the general quality of training of the other nursing staff. At the other extreme are the many homes that provide excellent care with loving attention paid to the physical, psychological and spiritual needs of the dying person.

It is clearly important to choose the right care home in the first place. Age Concern produce a checklist for what to look for in a home. For more information locally you can contact the National Care Standards Commission and you can find their number in the phone book. Others who may help are your social worker, GP or district nurse. A local hospice or specialist home care nurse may be able to tell you which homes they think provide good terminal care. You could ask each home the same questions as you would for a community hospital or private hospital. Add a simple question like 'Do sick residents have special food prepared or do they share the same menu as everyone else?' The answer may tell you a lot.

Choosing your hospital

It is impossible to predict how much choice you will have about which hospital or hospice you go to. The availability of beds varies from place to place and from time to time. For example, hospital beds are fuller during the winter than they are in the summer because of seasonally related disease. You only need a bad wintry fog to send patients with lung disease into hospital in their thousands. There will always be a bed in hospital if you need it, but if the local hospital is full patients occasionally have to be sent elsewhere. The length of time you may choose to stay in hospital is also primarily determined by the pressure on beds. If you are very ill and want to be in hospital you need not worry about this. Of course they will look after you. But if you are in hospital primarily for nursing care, and this is particularly true for the elderly, the hospital may discharge you to a nursing home without you having much option.

Assuming you are able to choose exactly where you are cared for, here are some considerations that might help you make the right decision for you.

- Where do you live in relation to the hospital? Most terminally ill patients go in and out of hospital several times during their last year, and they don't want the journey to be too onerous.
- Can visitors get to see you? Parking is sometimes awful in the city hospitals. Is there a bus or train? If so will the cost prohibit some of your friends from seeing you as much as you would like?
- What are the building and grounds like? It may be very important to you to see a few trees and enjoy the landscape. Can you get outside and enjoy fresh air and sunshine or is there nowhere to sit?

Within every hospital there is a great difference in the organization and structure of the wards. In older hospitals the general wards are still often Nightingale wards, long thin rooms with patients ranged down either wall and a nursing station near the door. Sometimes more than thirty patients are living in this one room, though increasingly wards are being made more tolerable by dividing them up into bays of six to eight patients. Life is then quieter, more private and more intimate.

All wards have side rooms. These are particularly important for a dying patient as they allow a degree of privacy that is impossible on the open ward. Visitors can sit all night with their loved one. They can make the space their own.

So, what kind of wards does your hospital have? Are they mixed or single sex? Which one will you be in and do you like it? Are there side rooms and if so how many? Ask the sister which patients generally use them.

Other patients

Fellow patients can be very important when you are in hospital. Intimate relationships develop tremendously quickly among patients in a bay or in the same area of a Nightingale ward. For some this can be a very positive reason for choosing to be in hospital.

But there is little privacy. Having your dressings changed, a catheter inserted, or your treatment and prognosis discussed behind curtains means that your neighbours will know all sorts of things about you that under normal circumstances you would never dream of sharing with family, let alone strangers. Does this appal you? Sometimes losing the usual means by which we preserve our dignity allows it to be redefined on a much deeper level. We all go to the toilet, we all smell, we are all capable of weeping in public, but we all pretend that we don't. To do these things in the sight of others can be perceived as undignified. But in hospital all patients are equally exposed. Breaching this dignity barrier is for many a liberating experience. The loneliness of your illness can be shared with other people who really understand because they are there too. Which is why the sight of one patient sitting by the bed of another comforting them after bad news or helping them through a painful or difficult time is so common and so moving.

But being with other patients can have its difficulties. It may upset you to see other patients getting better, leaving hospital to resume their normal lives. Sometimes, too, your situation may be distressing for those other patients—they feel unable to acknowledge what is happening to you and withdraw. You are left feeling very isolated.

A woman went to theatre for investigations and woke to be told she had an inoperable cancer. Her neighbours on the ward had all had hysterectomies for other conditions and soon began to recover. They came and chatted, asking her what she was in for. 'I just said I had had a hysterectomy too', she told me. 'I couldn't face their questions or their sympathy.' So her isolation in hospital was profound.

Dying remains for most people a very disturbing business. Patients in hospital already feel vulnerable and try to deny the possibility of dying. Staff collude with this denial. When a patient dies curtains are kept drawn around the bed until the body is to be moved. Then ward curtains are drawn around every bed so that no patient is disturbed by seeing the dead person leave. When the curtains are opened, the bed is empty as if by magic. Very rarely do staff talk to other patients about what has happened. It really is as if it didn't happen.

Compare this to a death I witnessed in a small hospital in Kenya. A young woman pregnant with twins had developed a condition known as eclampsia. Although the babies had been delivered by Caesarean the eclampsia continued. I was called to the maternity ward one evening because her condition had deteriorated. I arrived hot-foot with another English student to find that her heart had stopped and she was no longer breathing. Almost as a Pavlovian response my friend pulled the woman flat in the bed and started cardiac massage. But the patient's mother leant across her dead daughter and pushed my friend away. Then she stood and raising one arm above her head began to sing a hymn. Looking around I saw all the other young women on the ward standing by their beds in their pink hospital nightdresses, faces turned to the dead woman and singing with her mother. They faced her death and they bid her goodbye.

Patients sometimes need to be allowed to acknowledge the death of fellow patients and to say goodbye in some way.

Patients' relationships with staff

A fascinating study was carried out on a children's cancer ward some years ago. The children were asked to rank the staff in order of importance to them. Starting with the most important and ending with the least, here is the list they came up with:

the ward cleaner
the student nurse
the junior staff nurse
sister
the house doctor
the registrar
the consultant.

This was a study of children's attitude and as such reflects the realities of ward life very accurately. Adults would probably have given different answers influenced by what they knew of the medical hierarchy, but the children we can trust.

Every day the ward cleaner cleans your locker and around your bed, and if you want to chat she chats. She learns a bit about you and you about her. She doesn't have to do anything horrid to you, she doesn't have to deal with your illness, but she can grow fond of you and you of her. Student nurses can often find time to sit and get to know you, but sister has the ward to run so although she may bustle in and out she rarely has much time to spend with you. Meanwhile the doctors, at least the senior ones, are hardly ever seen. So when you think about your relationships with the staff make sure you think about them all. A warm sympathetic consultant is very important, but so too are the others.

In hospital you come into contact with many people who have some power over you. When you are ill you become dependent on others in ways that you would not have thought possible. Plus you are in your night clothes a lot of the time, dealing with fully fit adults who are also fully clothed. Should they choose to exercise their power you are in a very vulnerable position. Maybe the consultant keeps you waiting for three hours and then neither explains nor apologizes for the delay; or the porter chats up a nurse over your head while taking you to X-ray, as if you did not exist. As a patient you are constantly exposed and it is hard not to have your feelings hurt at some time by some act of thoughtlessness or lack of concern.

Medical and nursing staff are just like other people trying to deal with illness and death. Many find that their natural inclination is to run away from it. If they seem inept or uninterested it may be that they are out of their emotional depth. This is not an apology for medics, but it is another of the realities of hospital life. Staff invariably wish they could do better, and if they stopped to think for a minute they would realize how awful it is for the patient to feel avoided. But as a junior doctor or nurse you are busy, there is always something else to do first, and soon the day is over and you are tired and you promise yourself, 'I'll go and see how Mr Smith is tomorrow.' Patients who have been given bad news describe how previously friendly staff avert their eyes when hurrying past their bed. I know, because to my shame I too have hurried past many times. It has taken me years to learn to recognize my own fear of death and understand how it influences my behaviour towards patients. With time I have learnt that although taking the first step may still be difficult it is invariably rewarded.

Relationships between staff and carers

At home carers have a very central role in looking after their loved one and, as we have seen, it can sometimes be better for everyone if some of that role is taken on by the hospital. Hospitals have been rather inflexible institutions in the past. Once a patient was admitted they would insist on taking over all aspects of care and this sometimes had the devastating effect of marginalizing the carer. But it is my impression that hospitals are changing. Perhaps you get great pleasure from providing food for your loved one, from washing him tenderly or settling him down comfortably last thing at night. Nowadays I am sure the nursing staff will be delighted to accommodate your wish to share the care with them in this way. This fits well with the new philosophy of empowering patients and carers by encouraging them to share medical decision making with the professionals.

The hospital has a patient on whom all attention is focused and sometimes little heed is paid to the needs of his family. This is one of the problems that the hospice movement identified and set about addressing years ago. In a hospice the patient and his family are seen as a unit that must not be divided up and treated in isolation. Carer and patient are equally concerned for the other's welfare. If the needs of only part of this unit is looked after, the whole will suffer.

Little acts of thoughtfulness from the hospital staff are greatly appreciated by a carer, like someone stopping to ask how you are feeling or if there is any-thing that can be done for you. It would be unrealis-tic to hope that all the hospital staff will be able to empathize with your situation; however if just one person, perhaps the ward social worker, thinks about your needs, you may feel quite supported.

Problems can arise when the patient's family does not conform to the narrow definition of a set of parents and children or of immediate relations. Take the example of a gay woman who has lived for many years with her partner and her partner's child. Will the hospital be able to acknowledge them as a family? What if the patient has a group of friends he or she regards as family? It is sometimes difficult for the staff to recognize that this family is as important as blood relations to others. Christopher Spence, director of the Terrence Higgins Trust Lighthouse, wrote that 'claiming entitlement to our particular choice of family and insisting on respect for that choice is a basic human right.' It is your right to define your own family. If staff are to respect your choice, they may need to understand exactly who constitutes your family. If you talk to the ward sister at the beginning of your stay in hospital she can then explain to the other staff. It is very useful for medical staff to be able to differentiate your family from other friends and relations.

Communication between staff and carer can be fraught with difficulty. Firstly, it is often difficult to track down the senior doctor or nurse and when you do find them the conversation often takes place in the open ward or corridor and is rather rushed. Staff are becoming increasingly sensitive to these issues but still if you want more than a brief chat with a senior doctor there is no point trying to catch him on the hoof. You need to ask for an appointment to see him so that he can set some time aside for you. Secondly, there is the issue of confidentiality. In theory, at least, all information belongs to the patient first and the doctors should discuss anything with him before talking to the family. This is very difficult and as we know does not always work out this way. But it can further the feeling that you, the carer, are being marginalized.

Some decisions really should not be taken without your involvement. If there is talk of your loved one being discharged home you should always be fully consulted. You should also be involved in determining what services are being arranged for when you get home. The Community Care Act states that carers needs should be recognized and increasingly I think that they are.

Patients' feelings

Ask yourself what you can't do in hospital that you can at home. How important are these things and will they affect your decision about where you want to be cared for? You may lose several things that you value highly and these are some of them.

In hospital there is a very real loss of the physical comfort a carer or spouse can give. I heard the sad story of an acquaintance of mine who pulled the curtains around her dying husband's bed and hopped in to cuddle and hold him, bringing comfort to both of them. A nurse 'discovered' them and chastised them, implying that this was definitely unacceptable behaviour. I suspect that this attitude may be fairly universal, for very few hospitals make provisions for couples to sleep together or even to lie in each other's arms for a while.

Can you enjoy the food in hospital—is home cooking a pleasure that you can easily sacrifice? Of course, these days hospital food is much better than it used to be and you can always supplement it with food from home. For those who maintain an appetite, however, it may be an important consideration. The immense social pleasure afforded by sharing food with friends and family is also gone.

Can you see your dog or sit with your cat on your lap? The answer may be no, although in some imaginative hospices and hospitals there is now a pet visiting service. It may not seem like a big problem to those of us not attached to a pet, but can be for some.

What about the temperature in hospital? When I had a baby the temperature in the ward was very high and the air was dry and stale. I opened my window only to be ticked off by a midwife who briskly shut it. If you have a dry mouth or are short of breath it is very comforting to feel a cool breeze from an open window, but in hospital this may not be allowed. On the other hand, the cost of keeping a house warm all day long during the winter is considerable, and some elderly people have to stay cold. The enforced heat of a hospital is for them a great blessing.

If you have an acupuncturist, osteopath, aromatherapist or any other practitioner that does not fit within the rigid medical model you may be denied their help while in hospital, but you should cerainly ask, and ask as senior a person as you can—for example your consultant.

If you like to smoke or drink life is hard in hospital. You can join the corridor smoking gang if you are still mobile, but it is made into a rather sordid exercise. The great pleasure you might derive at home from lying back in your chair after supper and light-ing up is completely lost. You may be allowed a small alcoholic drink, but any hint of excess (as defined by the staff and not by you) will be frowned upon and probably forbidden. I don't recall ever seeing a bottle of wine gracing the patient's dinner table.

Cannabis is another drug that is much easier to take at home than in hospital as it remains illegal in the UK. Because it does have a therapeutic effect on a number of symptoms that are common in terminal illness I have discussed its use more fully on p. 203.

Most of all you lose the freedom to do what you like with your time. Life is ordered as I suppose it has to be, and that means that you are ordered. Meals are at set times, lights go out at the same time, and although you may be able to read or watch television quietly you generally have to fall into step with the ward routine.

How to make a decision

Both the patient's and carer's feelings are obviously important when it comes to making a choice about whether you want to be in hospital or not. Think clearly about how you feel in hospital. Can you bal-ance the positive against the negative and come to a decision about where you are best cared for?

What was the reason that you came into hospital? If it is to avoid being alone the decision is easy. If it is because you are suffering from symptoms that could not be satisfactorily controlled at home the main question is are they better controlled in hospi-tal? In general we know that symptom control is better in hospital than it is at home, but recent research has highlighted the difference in pain con-trol between wards in the same hospital. So for you

the important question here is how well your symptoms are being controlled now that you have come
into hospital. If you remain in pain, who is trying to
sort out the problem? If it is left to the houseman or
senior house officer and they are not succeeding you
need to ask someone more experienced for help. Ask
to see someone from the palliative care team if there
is one in your hospital.

Usually patient and carer agree that hospital is the
best place if nursing has become too difficult for the
carer at home. But I think people often come to this
decision with mixed feelings. The carer may feel
guilty, the patient resentful if both at heart believe
that home is the 'proper' place to die. There is no
proper place, so if you do have these feelings examine their origins and rethink. Perhaps your family has
always been cared for at home, and it seems unnatural to think of going to hospital. By implication you
are either weaker or less caring than those relatives
who have looked after their loved ones at home.
Perhaps your feelings arise from a fear of hospital that
has no rational basis. Is your image of hospital
coloured by a previous bad experience or have you
read or heard something that has prejudiced you
against them? One bad experience may not be truly
representative of the hospital care you are likely to
receive. Similarly, second-hand tales should be
reviewed critically—bad stories travel farther and
faster than good ones.

Problems arise when a carer feels unable to cope
but the patient really wants to stay at home. What
could make you feel more guilty or resentful than
that? If this should happen to you and your family,
make sure you talk to each other properly and aim to
understand each other's points of view. Can you

compromise? The patient might be able to go into hospital for a time to give the carer a rest (this is called respite care). Or someone else could perhaps step into the carer's role for a while. You must reach some agreement on this one or you are both in trouble. Anger and resentment may overtake all your good feelings towards one another. Maybe you need a third party to help you come to a decision—if so, who can arbitrate for you? You need someone that you both trust and who is impartial. Perhaps another member of your family could be brought into the discussion, or alternatively, you may need to turn to someone outside the family, such as your GP, hospital consultant or priest. Explain the problem and ask if they can help you resolve it. This will usually entail sitting down together and exploring both sides of the argument. Sometimes the problem can be resolved, sometimes it can't and one party will be left unhappy about the final decision, but at least you will know that you tried your best to resolve matters.

Maintaining a loving and mutually supportive relationship is tremendously important. If either of you are too tired, angry or resentful to be happy together at home, you need to change something and it may be the place of care. In the end you both need to know that you have done your best for each other. Doing your best does not always mean caring at home. Just because you do not care *for* a person does not mean that you do not care *about* them.

The hospice and palliative care services

Many of the problems associated with hospital care were recognized long ago and out of this awareness has grown the hospice movement. Hospices are built with the express purpose of supporting dying patients and their families, and as such the care they provide is significantly different from that available in a general hospital. They are the third important place in which terminal care is provided in Britain.

There is no doubt that most patients who are lucky enough to have contact with a hospice find that the care they receive there is of the highest quality. Today there are over 200 hospice and palliative care inpatient units in the UK, which between them provide 3222 beds. But of the 40 000 new patients admitted to these beds each year 96% are suffering from cancer, although they also take a few patients suffering from motor neuron disease or multiple sclerosis. There are some specialist hospices for patients with AIDS and there are some children's hospices. Otherwise, for the vast majority of patients who have not got cancer, no hospice care or its equivalent is available, which seems very hard. GPs and district nurses are constantly arguing with hospices about the unfairness of the system. Hospice staff reply that they are already swamped with work caring for patients with cancer and cannot open their doors to anyone else. Certainly their beds are constantly full and yet less than one cancer patient in five dies in a hospice.

This is a negative start to a discussion about one of the major advances in medical care in the second half of the twentieth century. My negativity is by way of an apology to all those patients who anticipated that their local hospice would be there to care for them, and who now find out that it is not.

There comes a time for many patients when there is no longer any point in striving to cure their disease, when further tests and treatments will do no good and may well do harm. In the old days a patient might have been told 'there is nothing more we can do'. But nowadays doctors do not stop looking after patients just because they cannot cure them. They recognize that it is equally important to continue actively treating all their symptoms so that they can live their life to its full potential even as they are dying. This is called palliation.

Palliative care is a term applied to a distinct medical specialty that has developed in the UK and all over the world during the last forty years. It has its roots in the modern hospice movement, founded in the 1960s by Dame Cicely Saunders. She drew her initial inspiration for the movement from a patient she met twenty years earlier when she was a young medical social worker. David Tasma was a forty-year-old Jewish man who came to England from the Warsaw ghetto; when Dame Cicely first met him he was dying of cancer. They talked, and from their talk arose the vision of a setting in which his symptoms could be controlled, but where there would also be space for him to find spiritual peace before he died. When David Tasma died he left a small legacy saying 'I will be a window in your home.' Dame Cicely took their idea and twenty years later founded St Christopher's Hospice in London. Since then the hospice movement has become established world wide.

The World Health Authority now recognizes this extended definition of palliative care:

- affirms life and regards dying as a normal process;
- neither hastens nor postpones death;
- provides relief from pain and other symptoms;
- integrates the psychological and spiritual aspects of care;

- offers a support system to help patients live as actively as possible until death;
- offers a support system to help the family cope during the patient's illness and in their own bereavement.

Most practitioners concerned with the care of dying patients should aim to provide care that is informed by these ideals. Whether at home, in hospital or in a hospice setting, the light from David Tasma's window illuminates the darkness far beyond the walls of St Christopher's Hospice.

It nevertheless remains true that the standard of care provided in hospices can not generally be matched elsewhere. Of course in individual cases this is not always true, but overall patients in a hospice receive better care than those at home or in hospital. Each hospice sets out to care for dying patients in a holistic way; it is central to their philosophy that the individual needs of each patient are considered in physical, emotional, social and spiritual terms. They also provide a high quality of service and this, of course, is expensive. Home care palliative nurses are similarly expensive, being highly trained with small case loads. Only by maintaining satisfactory levels of highly trained staff can they continue to provide a first-class service. Sadly, we cannot hope for such services to be expanded sufficiently to meet the huge need for this kind of care that exists within our society.

Palliative care services have, however, spread beyond the original inpatient hospices and can now be found in several different guises throughout the country. They are all free of charge regardless of whether they are funded voluntarily or by the NHS. Here is a summary of the main kinds of palliative care available. You need to find out which, if any, of these services will be available to you.

Hospices and palliative care units

Palliative inpatient care is provided in a number of settings, all offering the same kind of care. Inpatient means that there are beds in the hospice or special hospital unit for patients being looked after by a palliative care consultant. Each unit or centre has a different name according to who funds it and this can be confusing. There are:

- 161 voluntary hospice units across the country which are funded partly by local charities and partly by the NHS;
- fifty-seven NHS units which are built in NHS hospital grounds;
- ten Marie Curie centres;
- seven Sue Rider units that provide inpatient care specifically for patients with advanced cancer and others that provide some long stay, respite and terminal care for patients with other diseases.

In total this equals 235 units with 3222 beds between them. Approximately 29 000 deaths occurred in these units in the year 2000.

Day hospices

Day care is provided in many of the hospices that also have inpatient beds, but there are a growing number of units that provide day care only. These allow patients to continue living at home but have regular contact with the hospice. You might go once or twice a week and share social or creative activities with other patients. The chance to meet people in the same situation as yourself can be a great support. One woman said 'This is the only

time in the week when I can really be me.' Another
who wore a wig following chemotherapy found
that it was the only place that she felt happy not to
wear it.

There is usually also the chance to talk with your
specialist nurse or doctor who can review your
general progress. Treatment such as physiotherapy or occupational therapy, as well as hairdress-
ing, chiropody and beauty treatments may be
provided.

Specialist hospices

AIDS patients are the only group, other than those
with cancer, that have their own hospices. The
symptoms suffered by AIDS patients can be particularly severe, making care at home impossible for
some patients. The tremendous strength of support
for sufferers, particularly from the gay community
but also from many other sections of society, has
produced the will and the financial wherewithal to
provide these specialist hospices. They provide
AIDS patients with a compassionate environment
informed by hospice ideals.

There are several children's hospices that again
help their patients to live as fully as they can, protected from the anguish that such untimely death
provokes in others.

How do you feel about hospices?

You may feel ready to think about going to your local
hospice. You may be wearied by the battle against
your disease and feel that it is time to lay down your
arms and accept what is to be. But more likely someone else will suggest that you consider receiving care
from a hospice. This may be a terrible moment for

you. You are still fighting, still hoping to live. You do not feel ready to face death. For you hospice equals giving up, but hospices are not simply places you go to die. They treat terminally ill people helping them to a better quality of life and death. Just as in ordinary hospitals, patients come and go, and over half of all hospice patients eventually return home to die. For the fighters, here is the story of a patient who twelve years after first getting breast cancer is still doing battle.

Case history

Lizzie Deakin developed breast cancer when her youngest child was only two years old. She had surgery, radiotherapy and chemotherapy which left her with an ugly swelling called lymphoedema of one arm. In spite of becoming a single parent around this time she coped, always holding onto the hope that she was cured. Then eight years later the cancer came back in her hip bone. She had another operation and was given more radiotherapy. At this point her defences crumbled and she became severely depressed. 'I just wanted to curl up in a corner and die,' she said. She was seeing her GP once a week but the tranquillizers he gave her were no help.

Then her uncle and aunt suggested she contact a hospice. No one had suggested this before. Although the hospice was happy to look after her, the system demanded that her GP make a formal referral. When she asked him to do this he refused, saying that hospices were for people who were dying and that she needed to see a psychiatrist for her depression. She could not persuade him to make the referral and so in great distress she rang her father and asked for help. After he had spoken with the GP a referral was arranged.

Within two days she was visited by the hospice team and they arranged for her to come to their day club. She has now been going once a week for the last four years. It is a day when she does not have to put on her coping mask. She arrives at ten o'clock and is served coffee while she chats to the staff and other patients. Two nurses then come and speak privately to everyone, to find out what sort of week they have had and ask if anyone needs to see the doctor. If there are any problems the doctor is there to help sort them out. In effect, she has an open appointment with a specialist every week. Lizzie sometimes takes a bath and has her hair done. There is a religious service for those that want to go. And so the morning passes. At midday drinks are served as an aperitif, followed by a three course lunch. After this some people doze, read, knit or play scrabble, others walk in the lovely grounds. Various activities go on in the afternoon and currently Lizzie is learning to craft pewter. The day ends with a light tea before the hospice volunteers drive everyone home. For Lizzie it is like spending a day in what she describes as 'a little corner of heaven' with other patients who really understand how she feels. She says, 'The nursing staff are extremely kind and thoughtful and understanding, they give me so much love. They are as angels in disguise, nothing is too much trouble for them.' It is the best day of her week.

Admission to a hospice as an inpatient is generally for the same reasons as admission to hospital. You need treatment for symptoms that cannot be controlled at home or you need more nursing care than is available at home, either because you live alone or your carer is exhausted, ill or simply unable to cope with the amount of work. Perhaps you are much more comfortable being cared for in an institution.

You can also be transferred to a hospice or palliative care unit from a general hospital ward. If symptom control remains a problem in hospital, especially where there is no specialist palliative care nurse available, you should think about trying a hospice because they are most expert at managing difficult symptoms in terminal disease, and probably better than your hospital consultant or GP.

You and your family may need the holistic approach to care that the hospice provides, and you may not find this elsewhere.

Why choose a hospice?

Hospices are all about caring for dying patients and therefore some of the major problems of general hospital wards are avoided. Terminally ill patients are not marginalized and forgotten in the rush of the general ward. They are not 'difficult' patients from whom staff and other patients gradually withdraw. Because staff who choose to work in hospices do so precisely because they want to work with the dying, they turn towards you rather than away. They are interested in you and your family as people.

Extending care to the whole family unit is central to hospice philosophy, and many patients need to know that their carer is also being looked after if they are to find peace. For other patients the fact of death is so unstoppable and so wearying that the place of death is of little importance. They have turned their gaze inward as they draw away from life. But for the family the place and manner of death make a great difference to their experience of loss. Being welcomed and included by the hospice helps them later in the dark days of their bereavement.

If home is not the right place, a hospice is certainly the next place to turn if you want to keep some control over your death. The usual medical hierarchy of hospital is to some extent broken down in a hospice. Staff work as a team and though it would be untrue to say that no hierarchy operates, at least in theory all members are of equal worth. Patients and their families may be part of the team and will certainly be included in any decision making that affects their care.

Palliative care services are guided by a belief in openness. Patient and family cannot truly be part of the decision-making team unless all available information is shared. Consequently there is a problem for those patients who do not know their diagnosis and its implications; occasionally such a patient is admitted to a hospice but it is unusual. A relationship built on trust needs to be open from the beginning, and both carers and patients are given time to talk about their fears and regrets and hopes which can, of course, be enormously beneficial.

Yet a hospice is still an institution governed by rules and regulations with its own restrictive practices. Many of the restrictions that make hospital so much less attractive than home for a sick patient still apply to a hospice. Privacy, physical contact, choice of food, smoking, drinking and pets may all be restricted. You must ask your local unit about any particular concerns you have as each hospice will differ in what can and cannot be accommodated.

Recent research by Julia Lawton and published in a book called *The Dying Process* has highlighted two other areas of concern that you should be aware of. The first is that the hospice policy of openness extends even until the moment of death. Deaths are often allowed to take place in full view of other patients and not, as in hospital, behind drawn curtains. Julia

Lawton noted that it was at these times that the day room was particularly well used by other patients. The second is that even with the best treatment available a few people suffer very distressing deaths. As hospices have to prioritize patients according to their need, these deaths are more likely to take place in a hospice than elsewhere. At these times she described a feeling of general distress within the hospice in sharp contrast to the usual calm atmosphere.

Complementary medicine is practised in some hospices. Aromatherapists work regularly with patients and massage is often encouraged. In my local hospice one of the sisters gives very effective abdominal massage to constipated patients, others perform foot massage as a way of soothing and comforting anxious patients. Hospices have traditionally been associated with religious belief and some are still run by nuns. Certainly there is always a chaplain associated with each hospice, but the movement makes clear that care is freely available to people of all faiths or of no faith. I must say none of my Muslim patients has ever gone to a hospice, maybe because they do not think it is an option for them, and maybe because no one thinks to refer them. That most hospice patients are white and middle-class is a reflection of who chooses to use the service rather than who could use it. Perhaps you have grave reservations about an ethos that may be implicitly Christian (though not explicitly so); you could reassure yourself on this matter by discussing your concerns with the hospice staff.

The hospice staff welcome the chance to get to know you and your family and for this they need time. Not much time, but more than a couple of days. Sometimes patients are admitted and die very quickly, but on average people spend thirteen days in the peaceful and patient-centred atmosphere of the hospice. Many do get to know the staff and the ward by going in for a short stay earlier in their illness, perhaps to deal with symptom control or to have some respite care while their carer has a break. This means having the courage to think about the hospice before you necessarily feel that you are dying. If you can take this step you will reap many benefits and if you continue to live for many months or even years what will you have lost?

I have met many patients who have chosen not to go into a hospice, and nearly always that has been the right decision for them. But almost all my patients who have been cared for by the palliative care services have had only the highest praise for every aspect of their care.

Referrals to hospital and hospice

The mechanics of how your care may be shared by your GP, hospital and/or hospice are quite simple. Start with your GP. If you need to go into hospital either for medical treatment or for nursing care there are two ways she can organize it. If the matter is urgent, say your carer has fallen and broken her arm so there is temporarily no one to look after you at home, your GP will ring the local hospital and arrange for you to be admitted. Then she will ring for an ambulance which will take you into the hospital. If the matter is less urgent she can ring your consultant's secretary and arrange a bed for you in the next few days. Either your GP or the hospital will arrange transport for you if you need it.

You cannot refer yourself to hospital, although in desperation you can present yourself in casualty. But unless the staff there think you are an emergency they will send you home rather than admit you.

Referral to a hospice is different. Your GP will ring the hospice and arrange an admission for you. Admission may also be arranged by your hospital doctor or home care specialist nurse. Patients and their relatives can also refer themselves, though this is less common. Before they take you in, some hospice teams like to come and meet you at home and they will then arrange a bed for you. Where I work the hospice beds are in such demand that after this visit you may have to wait a week or more before they can admit you but it varies from hospice to hospice. Again, an ambulance or suitable transport will be arranged for you by the hospice.

If you are in hospital and would like to be transferred to a hospice the ward sister can usually make the arrangements for you and organize transport. Again you may have to wait some time for a bed to become available. Clearly where there is a palliative care ward attached to your hospital this process will be easier.

The sticking point is generally the queue for hospice beds. You cannot jump the queue even if you wanted to. The hospice staff try to take the most urgent cases first but, to be honest, it is impossible to say that one dying patient is more urgent than another. I have had patients who have died in the queue. It follows that if you want to be cared for by a hospice, delaying making the decision for too long may mean that you leave it too late for them to be able to help you.

4
Patients and Carers

I was leaving the flat of a ninety-two-year-old woman when her sister waylaid me in the hallway. 'Edith's had enough,' she said, 'she's just waiting for the call, but she knows there's nothing she can do to make it hurry up.' We then fell into conversation and I asked if Edith had been married. 'Oh yes, he was very good to her. She's had a lovely life you know, no kids, no worries, plenty of money.' I expect if you asked Edith about her life she might interpret events differently. But there was no denying that Edith was waiting for the call, she was weary of a life whose natural course had run far beyond three score years and ten. How different was she from the patient who has work still to do, commitments to meet, plans to see through, the patient whose biography has been interrupted by their illness. But whether young or old, weary of life or fighting to survive, everyone will wonder about the journey ahead and what it will hold for them. After ninety-two years my patient felt she was ready to find out.

In this chapter I consider many of the usual reactions and responses of both patients and carers to a terminal illness. Recognizing and working through some of these common anxieties and problems may help you to 'put your affairs in order' in a much broader sense than is generally supposed.

Patients' feelings

Patients who are 'ready for the call' seem to move easily into the sense of acceptance experienced by many dying patients. Their troubles fall away as they gently let go of life. They turn their thoughts ever inward and prepare to die. A time of serenity supervenes and anger, depression and anxiety are put behind them. For others the struggle with their illness is long and hard and miserable. It is fought to the last ounce of strength and will. There is no peaceful acceptance of death, only a weary admission of defeat.

Perhaps it is impossible to know what it feels like to be dying until it is happening to you. An American psychiatrist, Dr Elisabeth Kubler-Ross, decided she would listen to dying patients and try to understand how they felt. She worked in a Chicago hospital and there she started her now famous 'dying seminars'. She interviewed many patients and was able to identify several stages through which patients passed on their journey towards death. Often patients started with a period of denial, then became angry; they then moved into a bargaining phase followed by depression before finally achieving the peace afforded by acceptance. If I look at each of these stages individually you may find that you recognize some of your own feelings.

Although described as 'stages' Kubler-Ross recognized that most patients did not pass in an orderly way from one emotional state to the next. It is more complicated and more confusing than that. You may move quickly back and forth between them so that in the course of a day you have exhibited aspects of all five stages.

Denial

How often have I sat with a patient who asserts that no one ever told him what was wrong—yet I told him myself, or have it on good authority that he was told in hospital.

Case history

Mr Leach was a man with lung cancer who angrily waved his appointment letter from the radiotherapy department at me saying 'This is the first I knew about it, when I got this letter.' When he was in hospital the doctor had taken a small biopsy in order to confirm the diagnosis of cancer. Unfortunately a bacterium grew in the wound and so Mr Leach needed treatment for this infection. The doctor broke the news of the lung cancer to him, but ended the interview by prescribing antibiotics for the infection. Mr Leach latched onto the idea that he had been in hospital for a chest infection. He denied the news that he was not ready to hear. The letter told him again that he had cancer, and it seemed to him that he was hearing this for the first time.

Denial is a very important mechanism whereby we all protect ourselves from knowledge that we are not yet able to cope with. With time we assimilate the difficult information and our denial drops away. Often this is a gradual process. One day a patient talks about his illness rationally and with good understanding, the next he is to be found making elaborate plans for the future.

Occasionally patients deny their illness until the very end, but this is rare. Some manage to deny what they know to be true for months against all evidence to the contrary.

Case history

Mrs Williams had cancer with extensive bone secondaries. Her pain was severe and she needed high doses of morphine. 'How are you?' I would ask when I went to visit her. She would always reply 'Oh doctor, my arthritis is bad today.' Yet I knew that in hospital she had been told her diagnosis on several occasions. Finally, after months of this, I determined to sit with her and try to get her to talk about her illness, her fears, to connect with the real feelings that were lost under this cloak of denial. I sat there gently pushing her towards talking about how she felt about her pain, the morphine, her family and her future. She skilfully closed off all my open-ended questions, talking only about how she hoped that someone would find a cure for arthritis. 'Yes, it's one of the many diseases we need a cure for,' I said, but she was determined not to take up my challenge. She held onto her denial and would not let go. Eventually Mrs Williams became very weak and her family wanted her to go into the local hospice. Talking to the family afterwards I asked if she ever knew her diagnosis. 'Oh yes,' said her daughter, 'Dr Flowers told her over the phone just before she went into the hospice. I think that was a terrible way to tell her, don't you?' So finally she chose to hear, just as her life was slipping away.

All the doctors and nurses who looked after Mrs Williams were made very uncomfortable by her denial of her illness. It was hard to go along with the pretence of arthritis and yet we had to. But neither she nor her family shared our discomfort. Denying the illness helped them get through. It is interesting to reflect that doing so allowed Mrs Williams some control over her life. Finally, when she was ready, and not before, she took the decision to confront her approaching death.

This is quite different from the misery that can arise when the denial belongs to the carer and is not shared by the patient. Here is a story a priest told me about just such a case.

Case history

I was asked by a neighbour to call upon a woman who everyone knew to be seriously ill. On arrival the door was answered by her brother with whom she lived. I told him why I had come and he invited me in. He then told me that his sister did not know how ill she was and that I was not to tell her that she was dying or I would not be allowed to see her. I agreed.

We went to the bedroom and no sooner had he announced me than she said to me, 'I'm dying aren't I?' With what I thought was some presence of mind I replied, 'We've all got to die sometime haven't we?' But even as I spoke the brother had jumped on the bed of this emaciated woman and was shaking her, shouting 'You are not dying, you are not dying!' She looked at me helplessly as she said resignedly, 'All right.' I then told her we had been praying for her. She said that she was grateful for the thought but she did not now believe in God anymore. Before I could speak he was on the bed again shaking her and shouting 'Of course you believe in God, of course you do!' This time I felt under no restraint as I said, 'If she says she does not believe then she does not.' I will never forget the look of gratitude on that face flashing her thanks to me that someone at least was still treating her as an intelligent human being. I asked her if she would mind me praying for her as I still believed and she smiled and said 'No.' She then asked me if I would come again and I replied that I would be glad to.

Anger

With the awareness that you are going to die comes a terrible wave of anger. My patient brandishing his appointment letter was propelled straight into this stage.

Such anger is often unfocused and becomes irrationally directed at family, friends, professionals, even God. Often it begets an angry response because people understandably experience each assault as a personal insult. A colleague of mine described his sick mother rounding on her loving husband at a family meal. His crime was that he had forgotten to put out the salt and pepper. 'You're hopeless, hopeless, hopeless,' she shouted to the dismay of the assembled company, and she continued to berate him for several minutes. Surely she was voicing her despair: 'my life has become hopeless, hopeless, hopeless.' Yet this quite understandable feeling was expressed in anger and hostility towards the person with whom she felt safest.

The most dramatic and disturbing expression of anger erupted one day in a sixty-year-old bachelor.

Case history

Mr Myers had developed an inoperable cancer. My husband was his GP. He was called to the house because Mr Myers was said to be making a disturbance. On arrival he discovered his patient, whom he had always known as a quiet, self-contained man, completely smeared in honey. He was pounding honey and newspaper in a pot under the delusion that he was 'making a cake', raging and shouting, 'I've got to finish this cake.' He was distressed and could not be reasoned with. He had to be sedated and admitted to hospital.

Mr Myers had worked all his life in a menial job without praise or promotion, he had never married and had no friends. As far as we can tell he went mad when he realized that he was going to die. That was it. That lonely, narrow life was it. What would he leave behind, what memorial would stand for him when he was gone? His anger exploded into madness.

I tell this story because there is something in the wild extremity of his reaction that I can understand. We all share some of his feelings about the futility of life. Fortunately for most of us these are tempered by other, more positive feelings of achievement, of love given and received, a sense of our own worth.

Bargaining

It is clear that many people can influence the time at which they die. Kubler-Ross recounted many instances of patients making bargains with death or with God, along the lines of 'If you will just let me keep going until my grandaughter's wedding I will be a better Christian for the remaining days of my life.' 'Let me see my fortieth birthday, and in return I will be better and kinder to all around me.' Most of these bargains are made privately with God and need not be talked about aloud. They are another of the adjustments we make when drawing near to death. In their implicit acceptance of the inevitability of approaching death they may be the first sign you have of eventually arriving at a peaceful time when you are ready to let go of life.

Depression

Sadness, fear, misery, depression: we will experience many unhappy feelings when faced with our own death. So the first thing to say is that in terminal illness you can anticipate a period of depression during which time it seems there is no joy to be had in living. You may find that all your former appetites are lost, sleep is disturbed, you cry a lot, everything is hopeless. Many patients even think about suicide, especially in the early days when a terminal diagnosis has been made unexpectedly. This period of depression is part of the difficult journey that many dying people have to make. Terrible as it is, this suffering may be the route by which you come to terms with the new and unlooked for pattern of your life, and in doing so enter a final period of acceptance and peace. It seems hard to imagine, but depression can be turned to good account. It may be the means for resolving difficult and painful issues.

A central feature of depression is withdrawal into yourself, and this is very hard for your family and friends to bear. They want to have your old self with them for the last months of your life, to enjoy you, to comfort you. When depressed you are there but somehow not there—your depression is like a barrier between you and the world.

As a carer it is very difficult to know what to do. First try to accept that this is a normal reaction and try not to feel too angry with your loved one for feeling like this. Then stick with him emotionally. Let him talk and be prepared to listen without having to offer advice. Above all, try not to jolly him out of his sadness, for he has good reason to be sad. So have you, and you may find that you can share your sadness with him; he probably already knows or suspects how you feel. Don't be afraid that it will make him even more wretched, as talking about your own emotions may help reach him in his loneliness.

A caring GP or nurse will be prepared to take time to sit and listen with the patient, and may be able to encourage those who are reluctant to talk to open up a little. Some patients will always be happier not talking, and this must be respected. It is their way of coping.

Acceptance

When the playwright Dennis Potter was dying he gave a remarkable interview. In it he said, 'I grieve for my family and friends, and they are going through it more than I am.' His family and friends were still desperate to hold him back a little longer, to postpone the dreaded day when they would lose him. But he was ahead of them. He was getting ready to let go of life.

Case history

Keith Goodman was a young man who had a bone tumour and after a long and exhausting course of treatment he had a brief reprieve. Then within a few months his tumour recurred. He wrote in his diary 'I have to go all through this again. Come on cancer boy, you have to fight on.' That was in January. Within two months his fighting mood had changed and his mother said, 'He just settled in—he accepted the situation in March and recognized that he was not going to make it.' In his diary he wrote, 'The tide comes in and the tide ebbs, why can't I?' He accepted his death.

After patients have fought, raged, bargained and mourned for their lost life, many reach a peaceful time of acceptance. Much of it is spent sleeping, preparing for a longer sleep. Life is gently drawing to a close and there is nothing left to fight.

Where are you?

Do you recognize any of these responses as yours? Probably you have experienced and are still experiencing some of them. The fact that you are reading this book indicates that the period of denial is passing. You may still have days when it returns, as if to give you a break from the effort of constantly being aware of death. If this happens, then let it—you probably need some respite.

In Chapter 5 the difficulties that sometimes arise with prolonged and deep depression are discussed (pp. 166–167). But for most people there will be dark days of gloom and sadness, alternating with angry times and hopeful times. For throughout your illness hope may still exist, and so it should. Hope for a cure will be one of the dreams of most terminally ill patients. Later hope for a cure is replaced to an extent by the process of bargaining for extra time. With acceptance, perhaps, the last vestiges of hope are relinquished.

Positive experiences

In a questionnaire that I read every week in my Sunday paper, famous people are asked about themselves and one of the questions is 'How would you like to die?' Most answer, 'Suddenly in my sleep.' But I always feel that would mean missing out on one of the fundamental experiences of life. Life is for learning, and there is no doubt that many people learn a great deal very fast when they are dying. They learn about themselves—how they cope with pain, with fear, with loneliness. Some find huge and unsuspected reserves of strength and courage within. They find to their amazement that they can give comfort to their loved ones: 'If I am brave and conquer fear, you need not be afraid for me.'

Illness brings people together and this can be an unlooked-for joy. A book called *Living Proof; Courage in the Face of AIDS* celebrates the incredible ability of people to find good even in the midst of tragedy. Don Adler, who is HIV positive, writes, 'My mother and I didn't always get along. We had a relationship that was not grounded in the truth. About two years ago we confronted some very tough, very personal issues and stripped away all the lies. It was liberating to speak openly with her. We've spent the last few years building a relationship based on trust and encouragement. For the first time in my life I know she loves me.'

The love and support that is there waiting for you when you become ill are surely the most treasurable of gifts that you may ever receive. Dying, too, seems to open many people's eyes to the beauty of life. They see things for the last time and see them so clearly that it is as if they have never really seen them before. Dennis Potter described sitting at his window in the Forest of Dean desperately trying to finish his last play before he died. He looked out and saw the spring blossom on an old plum tree that he had seen flower many times before. Here is how he described his feelings: 'Instead of saying "oh, that's a nice blossom," now, last week, looking at it it's the whitest, frothiest blossomiest blossom that there ever could be, and I can see it. Things are both more trivial and more important than they were and the difference between the trivial and the important doesn't seem to matter. The nowness of everything is absolutely wondrous. If you see the present tense, boy do you see it and boy can you celebrate it.' Perhaps it is a gift given to the dying that they can see the present tense as no one else can.

Preoccupying problems

People who know they are dying have a lot of work to do if they are to leave their affairs in order. This work is both emotional and practical. Many of the decisions to be taken are ones that you will share with your carer but some are for you alone. As I have just said, some people can learn remarkably quickly when time is short and similarly some can achieve an enormous amount. You may have days when you are not well enough or strong enough to embark on any of these tasks so starting sooner rather than later can help.

Your dependants

Leaving behind the people we love is one of the most painful, tearing things that can be imagined. You are facing this. Yet while you are feeling your way through the huge questions of life and death, every-day matters will still be there, demanding attention. You find yourself ordering coal for the winter, filling the freezer, planning ahead as if in readiness for a time when you will not be there to do such things. Sometimes looking after practical matters can give a feeling of stability and continuity; sometimes it seems overwhelmingly sad. You will find your own way of working with and through these emotions. However difficult it may be, express your feelings to those you love so that you own the experience together and are not trapped in your separate griefs.

Your spouse

I use the word spouse to mean any partner. Time and time again I hear dying people express terrible anxiety about how their spouse will cope. This is a very real worry, for nearly all *will* suffer a painful bereavement, which is particularly acute for elderly couples who have lived together for many years. But most people can imagine the possibility of being happy again. You may be able to talk about this together. First think about how this makes you feel. One part of you probably wishes that your partner will grieve forever. A more generous side may understand that they can be happy and still remember you with love. Some bereaved people are helped if they are given permission by their dying spouse to be happy again in the future.

You can also support your spouse by considering practical matters. What do you need to teach him or her before you die in order that they may continue to function normally? Who knows about the running of the house? Who pays the bills? Who cooks and who cleans? It may be quite easy to sort out a lot of these problems that can cause more worry than they should. Of course during a long terminal illness the carer learns a good deal, but there may still be areas that you control exclusively.

Financial matters are of the utmost importance to your surviving spouse and clearly if you have made adequate provision for them there is no problem. Your solicitor, accountant or bank manager may need to know what is happening to you in order to advise you on sorting out your affairs.

Dependent parents

Dependent parents may preoccupy you. Telling parents what is happening to you is so difficult, for however old they are you are still their child. They feel they should change places with you, die instead of you, and of course everyone understands and to an extent shares this feeling. During a visit to an eighty-four-year-old man who was dying of cancer I was aware that he was not interested in his own disease. On the mantelpiece were several pictures of a middle-aged couple and their grown son. 'Ah, that's my daughter. She died two years ago of some sort of meningitis. She had an operation for two cysts in the brain and just when we thought she was getting better she got this meningitis. My grandson there is a good boy, but he can't get over to see me much because he works in Birmingham. Mind you, he comes home every night to be with his dad, keep him company. He started that after his Mum died.' He was uninterested in his own health because he was still grieving for his daughter who was only sixty-one when she died. The Compassionate Friends is a nationwide befriending organization which offers support to those who have lost a child, of any age. The address is on p. 237.

Dependent children

The pain of leaving young children is so terrible that sometimes parents cannot face talking to their children about what is happening. This has been explored a little in Chapter 1. However you choose to approach this, you need to remember that you will remain one of the most significant people in the rest of their lives. Talking to them and telling them how much you love them, sharing your sorrow with them, particularly your sorrow at leaving them, is probably the most important gift you can give them. It may be too much for you to bear. You may be clinging to hope so hard that you do not want to even glimpse the possibility of their life without you. Perhaps another person needs to help you: your spouse, a family friend that you really trust, or a professional such as your GP, nurse or social worker. If you have contact with a hospice there will be someone there for you, whether social worker, chaplain or medical staff. Ask for help, for it is perhaps the most difficult thing that you have to do.

You will need the help of a lawyer or of social services if you are a single parent. Planning ahead for the children sometimes involves making extremely difficult decisions about legal guardianship. If your children are to be adopted you may be able to meet their new family, to send them with your blessing.

Extended families

As a result of remarriage following death, separation or divorce, many families have become rather complicated groups involving step parents and children and half brothers and sisters. The potential for conflict in any family is heightened by the inevitable stress of caring for someone who is terminally ill but in these complicated families things can often be just a little more difficult than usual. Who controls access to the ill person, who makes decisions about how and where they should be looked after? Who is in charge of funeral arrangements and even who is the next of kin? These are a few of the many potential areas for conflict.

In my experience families function most harmoniously when it is clear to everyone that the person who is ill is actually making their own decisions.

When you are ill this may be quite difficult and exhausting. But it really helps still the anxiety of family members who for one reason or another are not able to fully trust each other. You may need to be explicit, for example say 'I am in hospital because I want to be, not because of anyone else' or 'I'm sorry that I can't always speak to you when you phone but I get very tired. That's when I ask my partner to take my calls and she passes your message on.' Most anxiety arises when people who love you fear that you are not getting the care you need. Letting them know that you are getting the care you want will certainly reassure them.

Leaving gifts

What are you going to leave behind for your family to help them remember you? These days they can hope for more than just a faded old black and white photo. Throughout her adolescence a great friend of mine watched her mother slowly dying. They were a loving and open family who coped remarkably well with this protracted and untimely death. Six months after her mother's death Susie came upon a book that she had been writing. She describes desperately snatching it up, hoping to find some reference to herself and her mother's love for her. Instead she found it was a novel about being in hospital, which made no mention of her family. It was a bitter blow.

That was twenty years ago when no one thought about leaving gifts for their children. Arising from work with parents dying of AIDS, Barnardos has produced a wonderful box called a 'memory store'. They realized that it was vital to build up a family history for children who were facing separation from a parent. Such a history allows children to know directly from their parent about themselves, their family, and the most important events in their lives. One of the overwhelming tragedies of AIDS is that if one parent is affected the other may be too, and so the 'memory store' is especially adapted for children who become orphaned. The store is a brightly coloured box the size of an attaché case. It includes drawers for small keepsakes, space for a video of family events and recordings of the parent's voice. There is a memory book for parents to record essential information, with space for addresses, photos, maps and a family tree. There is also an explanatory booklet. If you would like to find out more about this it is listed in the useful addresses section on p. 227.

Most people can adapt this idea to suit their own needs. You could buy a beautiful wooden box and fill it with things that have been important in your life together. Any record of life is valuable whether it be something that you have written for your child or a video or a tape recording of your voice. There will come a time when your children will want to look, want to hear your voice or read your words. It may be too painful for a long time but there is no hurry— your box can wait for them.

Making a memory store need not be a solitary occupation and indeed some people make it together with their loved one. One woman described how she took her favourite scarf and put it in the box after letting her daughter hold it, smell it and rub it against her cheek. They both understood that if her daughter needed to sense the nearness of her mother, she could again hold and smell and bury her face in the scarf.

As a society we are increasingly keeping photographic records of significant events in our lives.

This is beginning to extend to the dying process. Gill Walkey, a friend of mine with cancer said 'I know I must be dying because everyone keeps taking photographs of me.' Her family and friends want a record of what may well be her last Christmas, birthday or holiday. Gill says she knows why they are doing it but laughingly adds 'Sometimes I feel like saying for God sake stop!.' David Lunn and his wife Rosie took a different approach and actively compiled a photograph album recording David's death. He had developed an inoperable bowel cancer in his fifties and died within a few months of the diagnosis being made. In those months he posed for a formal family portrait and there are informal pictures of him with Rosie and with his children, family and friends. Towards the end there are pictures of him sitting up in bed with his son and daughter leaning against him. The day of his death, which was a beautiful snowy February day with bright sunshine streaming into his room, is recorded with David asleep and his family all around. In one of these pictures they are eating pizza and drinking wine, which is a bit shocking but actually forms part of a true record of the day. The final picture is a peaceful photograph of David after he had died. It is surrounded in the album by dried flowers.

Rosie had a friend whose husband had also died when his children were young. Years later the children said they regretted not being able to remember what his death had been like. It was because of this that Rosie and David made the album. Rosie says 'We did it to remember. However unbearable it was at the time it was done to remember.'

A patient I was treating for depression after his wife died, came to me after the first anniversary of her death. He said 'Last week I got out all the old cine film of Rose and me, you know, down at the caravan, in the garden and things. I sat and edited it all day Sunday. Tears were streaming down my face all the time, but I did it.' He did it with great difficulty but it was very important to him to be able to look at her again as she was when she was alive and happy. It was a sign that he was beginning to turn a corner and start to come out of his depression. Very few people are photographed towards the end of their life. We generally do not think of recording images of ourselves when we are tired or ill. Yet these very images can bring comfort to family and friends later on, they help them remember you as you were, for they have loved you when you were ill just as much as when you were well.

Unfinished business

Many people come to the end of their life with unfinished business. Should you have such business the question is do you want to finish it before you die? Estrangements within the family are very common. The enormity of what is happening to you can often make former arguments and feuds pale into relative insignificance. Now can be a time of reconciliation, of healing and coming together. If, however, you attempt a reconciliation only to be rejected this is sometimes more than you can bear when you are weak and ill. You may be too angry to contemplate any form of reconciliation, and may yourself reject overtures made towards you. Perhaps you may feel differently later on in your illness, so take time to think about these things.

Secrets

We all have secrets; some are so private that we have hidden them away for much of our life. What are you going to do about them now?

There may be secrets from your past that you have hidden from your family. Perhaps, for example, you have a secret criminal record, or you had an illegitimate child who was adopted years ago. Perhaps you have had an affair or been secretly bisexual or homosexual. Can this remain your secret forever or will your family find out about it when you are no longer around to protect them? If they are certain to find out then it is kinder and braver for you to tell them. They may understand and find it easy to forgive you. They will certainly not think the worse of you for telling them. But if they find out too late they may never be able to satisfy their need to understand what went on. It takes great courage to break the silence of years, but for some the fact of their dying gives them unlooked for strength in all sorts of ways.

There are other secrets that will certainly be revealed. What if your financial affairs are in a mess? For people who have always prided themselves in running their affairs efficiently this may be a shameful thing and it demands courage to face your family and tell them what has gone wrong. There may be an explanation you can give that will help them understand.

Love affairs may also be very complicated and distressing, especially if they are ongoing at the time of your illness. At the best of times they occasion complicated and divided loyalties which now intensify: loyalty to your spouse who has been faithful and loving all your life and whom you cannot bear to hurt;

loyalty to your lover who faces a particularly bitter and lonely bereavement. I remember a middle-aged woman overwhelmed with grief at the impending death of her lover of twenty years. She had clung to the hope that one day he would leave his wife and marry her. Now he was dying and that dream was dying with him. She felt she had been duped out of her youth, waiting all this time for nothing, not even a place at his funeral. Another young woman described her lonely bereavement through tears; her affair had been so secret that no one knew. She continued working and living outwardly as if nothing had changed and yet inwardly she was crushed with grief. Not saying goodbye, choosing not to be the mysterious woman at the back of the funeral crowd, was for her the bravest and most painful part of all. These women were both disenfranchised grievers, their bereavement unrecognized by society.

If you too are in this position say goodbye to your lover properly while you still can. If you need to continue to see both your spouse and your lover think about going into hospital rather than spending all your last days at home. Explain your dilemma to a sympathetic member of staff and it may be possible to arrange for you to keep your secret and still say your goodbyes. It will not be the first nor the last time that it has happened.

Legal matters

There are several different kinds of legal business that you may wish to deal with.

Your will

Only one in three adults in Britain have a will, and yet almost everyone knows that dying intestate causes great problems for relatives and loved ones.

If no will has been made the intestacy rules dictate who will inherit and manage the affairs of your estate, who will be your legal representatives, and who will be the legal guardians of your children. In English law an unmarried partner may not have any rights of inheritance.

Making a will can be expensive but a reasonably straightforward will generally costs about £50. Contact a solicitor if you want to be sure that your will is going to be legally watertight. If you are too ill to go to them they will come to you. Some people draw up their own wills. If you favour this you can be guided by The Law Society leaflet 'Ten Steps to Make a Will' or contact Age Concern who offer a cheaper will-making service.

It is possible to take satisfaction in making your will, cannily minimizing the Inland Revenue's cut from your estate, planning what special bequests you want to make to friends and family. Making a will or altering a will for the last time is all part of the process of letting go—letting go of both the responsibilities and the physical trappings of your world.

Power of attorney

There may come a time when you are no longer physically capable of ordering your own affairs. In preparation for this you can nominate someone else to act on your behalf. You give them power of attorney over your affairs. You can revoke this at any time. Enduring power of attorney is different as it continues regardless of your mental ability to manage your own affairs. It may be useful in several circumstances. For example, an elderly woman developed Alzheimer's disease and became incapable of living alone. Clearly she needed to go into a nursing home and fortunately her niece had been given enduring power of attorney over her affairs. Her niece was therefore able to raise money for her care, initially by cashing in her shares and later on by selling her house. Without this power the elderly woman would have been placed in a cheaper home (even though she was wealthy) because her assets were all tied up. With her money released she could live in a much more expensive and infinitely preferable home, with a room of her own and a view of the hills.

Living wills

Living wills are also called 'advance directives' and they are now appearing in Britain having been in use in the United States for some time. A living will is a document which allows you to continue to exert control over your treatment if you become mentally or physically incapable of discussing matters with your doctors and carers. It provides instructions to both doctors and relatives who may be faced with making very difficult decisions on your behalf. The will also ensures that you are treated as you would wish. Quite often patients reach a time when they are ready to die, but their family are unable to let go. Rather than face the finality of death, relatives urge doctors to 'do everything they can'. In such circumstances a living will written together with the carer's knowledge and approval may help guide everyone concerned through this most difficult of times. The same is true for patients in residential or nursing homes where staff may feel that they must be seen to have done everything, which is not always in the best interest of the patient. Neither staff nor relatives feel confident to take the decision not to treat.

What sort of treatment do living wills commonly deal with? With a terminal illness they become relevant only if you are unable to participate fully in decisions involving your medical care. You can state that in such a circumstance you do not wish any treatment to be given aimed specifically at prolonging or sustaining your life. You can then expand accordingly. For example, you might say that you wish all distressing symptoms to be treated but would not want to be kept alive by 'artificial means'. In effect this means that your GP would withhold antibiotics if you developed a chest infection, anaemia would not be treated with a blood transfusion, but morphine could be given for pain relief. Several variations on the basic document are available. The Terrence Higgins Trust Lighthouse has produced one for patients with AIDS because AIDS dementia is common. The Voluntary Euthanasia Society also produce one which has been adapted sensibly by the Natural Death Centre (see p. 228).

The British Medical Association advises that you discuss the will fully with your doctor, put a copy in your medical notes and carry a card that says that you have made one. In 1994, in a reply to a parliamentary question, the Prime Minister said:

Her Majesty's government acknowledges the right of individuals to draw up advance directives. People have a right, emphasized in the Patient's Charter, to consent or withhold consent to treatment. Advance directives assist patients in the exercise of their legal rights and so ensure their lawful treatment.

As a GP I have not yet had a patient who has made a living will. In Britain, on the whole, there is a relationship of trust between the medical profession and terminally ill patients. It is no coincidence that living wills are more common in the United States which operates a system of private medical care. It is somewhat harder to trust your doctor to withhold treatment when it is in his financial interest to continue.

What we do not always do very well in Britain is to recognize the importance of sharing decisions with patients, and encouraging real co-operation between patient and doctor when it comes to planning care. If you have strong feelings about the kind of treatment you would or would not like why not go and talk to your GP about it? Most GPs would be very excited if you offered to share some of the difficult decisions with them.

Euthanasia

In 1994 the House of Lords Select Committee on Medical Ethics defined euthanasia as 'A deliberate intervention undertaken with the express intention of ending a life to relieve intractable suffering'. This is different from withholding or withdrawing treatment necessary to the continuation of a person's life. It is also different from the appropriate use of drugs to control or relieve symptoms that may result in the hastening of death. These are both legal actions. In the final chapter of this book there is an example of a patient who died while her GP was giving her an injection of diamorphine to relieve her pain. Although this may seem like euthanasia it is not. The GP's actions were perfectly legal as he was giving the drug to relieve his patient's symptoms even though her death was probably hastened as a consequence. This is known as the 'double effect'.

The select committee concluded that 'There is not sufficient reason to weaken society's prohibition of intentional killing which is the cornerstone of law and of social relationships.' So euthanasia remains illegal.

As with other controversial debates, attitudes to euthanasia are polarized. About a quarter of the population advocate euthanasia on demand and another quarter will not contemplate it under any circumstances.

What about doctors? At least half of them have been asked to take active steps to hasten a death at some time in their career. A third of these (i.e. a sixth of all doctors) have complied. In a survey of GPs two out of three said they would not comply with such a request. Surprisingly, it was hard to predict which GPs would comply and which would not. Roman Catholics were equally spread across the two groups.

Perhaps it is easier to have a clearly held opinion on the rights or wrongs of the matter when you are not involved with a patient who is facing death. Once embroiled in the emotional welter of terminal illness certainties are often replaced by ambivalent feelings. Mr Reed cared for his sick wife Anne for many years. They had talked to me and the partners in my practice about her wish to die and we had all agreed to withhold life-prolonging treatment. None of us offered euthanasia. It was only recently, after her death, that Mr Reed told me that they had seriously considered going to the Netherlands where euthanasia is practised openly. In the end this went no further than talk. Anne eventually fell into a coma. Her husband delayed calling an ambulance for two hours but then realizing she was not going to come round rushed her into hospital where she died half an hour later. He said to me, 'Sometimes I think to myself, if only I had called the ambulance earlier she might have lived a little longer.'

Some will view euthanasia as a kind of rational suicide, where the decision to end a life to shorten suffering is shared between patient and physician. Of course there is a powerful prohibition against suicide in our society, which partly at least derives from the Christian tradition. In a sense, therefore, if a patient and physician share this most difficult of decisions they also share the responsibility for what follows. Thus for many patients euthanasia is acceptable whereas suicide is not. When Mr Reed told me about his Netherlands discussions I asked if he and Anne had ever considered suicide to which he replied, 'I don't know, you know, we never thought of it, I suppose.'

It is worth noting that although euthanasia is practised in the Netherlands they will not accept 'euthanasia tourists', that is people like Mrs Reed who want to go there in order to die. The best book that I know on the subject is *Dancing with Mister D* by Bert Kaiser, a Dutch doctor who practices euthanasia and I recommend it to anyone who wants to know more about the Dutch way of death. For more information on both living wills and voluntary euthanasia or physician-assisted suicide contact The Voluntary Euthanasia Society (UK) or Exit—The Voluntary Euthanasia Society of Scotland (see p. 229 and p. 226 for details).

Shared concerns of patient and carer

Dividing the concerns of patient and carer is rather contrived. I have not written in this way with the intention of excluding one or other of you from any of the considerations discussed in this chapter. Some matters are obviously shared concerns and in the following section I will consider these before turning specifically to matters affecting carers.

Practical matters

Financial concerns are clearly shared concerns. Planning for the future is one of the great worries that some patients and carers can allay by working together, anticipating problems and setting wheels in motion to prevent future hardship. Making a will is clearly of great significance to a spouse, and I would expect most couples to sit down together when drawing one up. I have written about wills under patient concerns because there may be no financially dependent carer.

Making a file of all important documents and addresses can save a great deal of searching and panicking later. Bank account numbers, building society address, solicitor's address, life insurance details, debts and loans, share certificates. Your bank accounts may be frozen on your death and so putting them into joint names at this stage may avoid your spouse temporarily being without access to money.

Pregnant mothers often make a birth plan in which they state the kind of delivery they want. They stipulate whether the baby will be born at home or in hospital, what sort of pain relief the mother would like, and so on and so forth. Some patients like to think about where and how they would like to die in rather the same way: the place, the atmosphere, the sounds and smells, who they would like to have with them and what should happen to their body afterwards.

The funeral

A priest told me it was remarkable how often when he asks a bereaved family what kind of funeral or cremation their loved one had wanted, they turn to one another blankly and confess that they have no idea, no one ever asked. At the other extreme, some people acknowledge the importance of the funeral ceremony by helping to plan their own funerals; choosing the celebrant, the place, the readings and music. Maybe you find this all distasteful, much too difficult and painful to think about. Yet just as death is inevitable for all of us, so is a funeral. It is something you and your carers might want to think about. Even the briefest of discussions may help carers feel happier about the kind of funeral they eventually arrange. Carers, family and friends all need to feel that the funeral is a fitting memorial to their loved one.

In the book *Funerals and How to Improve Them* by Dr Tony Walter, he says this about the contemporary funeral: 'Within a century, we have swung away from showy funerals that went way over the top in displaying social status, to plastic funerals that say nothing, that say the person was nothing. No wonder some people would rather do without a funeral altogether. No wonder the funeral has become an ordeal to be endured. And yet some funerals are not like this. Some mark the passing of a human life with sorrow but also with integrity. Some offer a chance to say goodbye. Some manage to say what is unsayable … A funeral provides an opportunity publicly to mark the passing of a human life. All too often we waste this opportunity.'

A useful book is *Funerals, a Guide* (see p. 241 for details). It is a collection of appropriate prayers, readings and music drawn from a variety of cultural traditions, especially the Christian heritage. The meaning and significance of the customary funeral service is explained and variations upon it and alternative forms are suggested.

Case history

Katy Frankish was an extraordinary girl who at the age of thirteen faced death square on. She used her final weeks both to celebrate her life and at the same time to prepare for her death. Not only did she prepare herself but she helped prepare her family and friends. This included planning her funeral arrangements. She chose a simple coffin supplied by the alternative funeral directors Heaven on Earth in Bristol which she decided would be painted sky blue. After she died her friends and family came and decorated it. They painted hearts, flowers, birds and butterflies on the outside and put pictures, poems and messages inside. As they were doing this they talked and thought about her. The process of decorating her coffin was both an expression of love and a tribute to Katy. It was one of the many ways in which she helped others to face up to the unbearable thing that was happening to her.

If you want to explore some of the less common funeral options *The New Natural Death Handbook* talks about these in some detail, and the Natural Death Centre will advise on how to organize a 'green' funeral.

Your relationship

How is your relationship going to stand up to the trial ahead? This will depend a great deal on what it was like before, for an open loving relationship will probably stay open and loving, while more difficult relationships will struggle more. Encouragingly, one study of patients with cancer showed that in most cases relationships with spouses were likely to have changed for the better. Patients and carers often rise to the occasion, proving themselves more courageous and stronger than either of them had suspected. Some relationships are nevertheless put under great stress with little empathy existing between partners. It may help to understand the kinds of feelings— both positive and negative—normally experienced by patients and carers.

Changing roles

In most relationships different roles are assumed which are partly defined by and in turn define the power structure within the relationship. Over time roles gradually mutate; so, for example, the power structure within a father/daughter relationship shifts as she reaches maturity and leaves home. This is usu- ally a gradual process. In spite of the daughter's inde- pendence some vestige of her childhood dependency remains in her relationship with her father. When he becomes ill and she becomes his carer their relation- ship may be transformed overnight, as she becomes the powerful provider and he the receiver of care.

Although illness may shift the power structure within a relationship, it is by no means clear in what direction it will move. The power of the patient may be enhanced as he lies in his bed with everyone running around looking after him.

Which way has power shifted within your relationship and is it a comfortable shift for both of you? A drastic shift or complete reversal of roles can often be very painful and lead to great resent- ment. The woman who has always prided herself on running a house and family and working too will find that her illness completely strips her of many of these cherished roles. Having to rely on others to keep the house clean or look after the children can be heartbreakingly difficult. 'I can't stand the mess in the house, no one ever seems to clean it up and I can't. It makes me so mad with them.' The mess makes her angry, it is frustrating not to be able to sort it out herself, but what makes the patient really mad is that it is her illness that has put her in this helpless position. Her negative feelings are expressed in rage directed at her family for not clearing up. Many patients and their carers say 'it's not like me to be like this' and that is really the point. You can become 'not like you' as a result of all the new pressures you find yourself under.

Loss of income is a major blow for dying patients and their families and one that we consider in practical terms on pp. 219–222. The loss of the status associated with work can be devastating, as we see in any family hit by unemployment. And it is boring being at home all day. The effects are actually so profound that death rates rise among the unemployed and no one really has a satisfactory explanation for this.

Unemployment due to illness can lead to another type of role reversal. The family breadwinner may change and this may be a source of immense resentment in a family where roles have hitherto been strictly defined. Carers are often forced to give up their own work in order to dedicate sufficient time to caring for their loved one. This too can be a devastating loss.

If your relationship sits quite peacefully with its new roles you are lucky. If it is uncomfortable, try to think about which elements are particularly distressing. Perhaps you can change things a little in favour of your old ways. A sick mother can be encouraged to plan the family meals or order the cleaning of the house to her own satisfaction. A grandmother's role as treater of the children might be preserved by arranging for them to have a regular trip to the sweet shop which she finances.

Sexuality

Just as no one used to think about the sexual desires and difficulties experienced by disabled people, so today the problems of the very ill are often brushed aside.

What are the common problems? They divide into those associated with desire and those associated with function. If you have had a fulfilling sexual relationship prior to your illness you may be facing a profound sense of loss. Feeling tired or ill, depressed or angry will all crush sexual desire, and both carer and loved one may be affected. Changes in your body as a result of your illness may make you ashamed, even horrified at the thought of making love. The disease that is particularly associated with these feelings is breast cancer. Up to a third of patients who have a mastectomy find that love making is difficult after the operation and many cease to make love at all. Time spent after the operation in some form of counselling—with nurse specialist or counsellor— can help some couples to accept what has happened and to rediscover their lost sexuality. Many other diseases are equally as distressing. Profound weight loss, hair loss, loss of function caused by a stroke, multiple sclerosis or motor neuron disease, are all a challenge. Not only do they affect the sufferer but of course their partner responds to these changes too. Carers often feel ashamed that they lose their desire, that they may even feel revolted at what is happening to the body of their loved one.

I like the story of the husband who gradually encourages his wife to look at her mastectomy scar, who mourns with her for the loss of her beautiful breast, but who continues to desire her sexually and gradually persuades her that she too can feel sexual desire again. It is the recognition and understanding of the loss that is important. So often it is easier either to pretend that these feelings aren't there, or to feel so overwhelmed that you turn away emotionally and physically from your loved one. This turning away reinforces their feeling of being 'diseased'.

There *are* physical problems that must be overcome if you are to preserve your sex life. Problems with mobility and flexibility, problems with pain, problems with impotence. You need to work out gently what is best for you. It is surprising what physical difficulties can be overcome. For example, a man can still have sexual intercourse with a urinary catheter coming out of his penis by using an ordinary condom to strap the tube back. Having a colostomy need not stop you making love. You may need some help initially and either the district nurse or a specialist nurse can advise you. Alternatively you can ring the British Colostomy Association or the incontinence nurse for your area and they can advise you over the phone. It may be embarrassing to talk about but it is a normal and very important part of life.

The wife of a man with motor neuron disease talked very movingly about the gradual change his disease brought to their love life. 'I think that as his desire lessened so did mine too, we were in harmony really. Later I flirted with him outrageously every evening when I got him ready for bed and it was great fun. We both enjoyed it enormously.' Sexuality exists without sexual intercourse, and you can give pleasure to each other in many ways. There is great pleasure in comforting physical contact for itself, to stroke, to massage, to lie in one another's arms. When one of you is disfigured by a disease this becomes particularly important. Acknowledge your loss, acknowledge your difficulties. Both of you are upset by these things. To be able to comfort each other physically is the ultimate way of affirming that it is the disease and not the person who is unattractive.

With the spread of AIDS the sexual problems of the dying have taken on another dimension. How can you be sexually active when it involves exposing your partner to a fatal disease? Studies show that provided a condom is used consistently there is minimal risk, and indeed I have looked after several couples who have chosen to go down this road and trust the research. The level of dedication both have to each other and to the maintenance of their sexual relationship have always seemed remarkable to me. With an open, honest relationship these most difficult decisions can be made. The importance of the sexual relationship to many couples cannot be better illustrated.

Family matters

For parents of dependent children probably the most important matter to think about together is how to maintain some kind of normal family life. How are you going to organize the family? Over half the parents who develop cancer are unable to care for their children as much as they did before and clearly the same is true of many other diseases. Carers of relatives or friends who are ill may also have young children in the house to look after.

You will probably need more help with the children, either from relatives or friends. School needs to know about the situation as your child's work may suffer, and schools can be very supportive to the child. Social services may be able to help by providing temporary nursery places or a mother's help at least some of the time.

It is important to the children that some sort of normality is maintained amidst all the change and the fear. Can you establish a new routine that includes them? Watching television together after school may provide a regular comforting family hour and they will not mind if you doze off as long as you are there. Perhaps one family meal a day can be preserved, which might simply be fruit and sandwiches taken in the patient's room. In my family this is called a monkey's supper, and it is particularly good if the children have had a hot school meal during the day. Children are often denied a useful role within the family until they are quite old. Although it is necessary to protect them from some aspects of the illness, they can nevertheless be given really useful jobs to do. Tailor them appropriately and make them part of the loving care their parent needs. Don't expect them to keep their bedroom tidy any more than you usually would. Providing fresh flowers twice a week for a sick parent to enjoy, or helping brush the parent's hair every morning when doing their own, remembering to bring the evening newspaper home after school or even taking turns to plan and make the monkey's supper every night. Children can enjoy doing these things and they will appreciate the chance to be involved in a useful way.

Carers' concerns

Feelings, like the protagonists in old westerns, are easily cast as good or bad. We allow our good feelings but we are frightened and ashamed of our bad ones. Just as a mother cradling her new baby, filled with love and tenderness, will hardly believe the anxious, helpless and angry feelings that same baby is soon bound to provoke in her, so a loving carer cannot at first believe the bad feelings that will almost certainly be experienced.

Good feelings

Alison Cornford cared for her mother at home during her terminal illness (described in Chapter 6). Several years later she said this of the experience: 'Mummy really gave me something by allowing me to care for her. She gave me so much back. She acknowledged my mothering of her. It was a great privilege and a very precious thing to be allowed to look after her at home.' The caring role is indeed very precious. Carers are rightly proud of themselves, especially when their care has resulted in a good death. Carers display a host of good qualities: love, loyalty, steadfastness, unselfishness, organizational skill, sensitivity, strength. For Alison Cornford the wonderful thing was that her mother acknowledged her mothering role. This is so important. Carers need recognition of their role and its difficulties.

Caring for someone at home can bring a profound sense of achievement. Mrs Jenkins who was so terrified about caring for her husband at home (see Chapter 2) was able to look back afterwards and feel proud. She had been incredibly brave, she recognized her fear and yet she overcame it. There is a sense of having done the right thing, proved something about yourself, recognized your strength. You may also recognize special gifts or skills that you possess. Another carer said, 'One of the things that I did was to let

Atilio be in agony, be sad.' She allowed him his emotional pain, and she was proud of the strength this revealed within her. There is the honour of being chosen as the carer, showing that you are thought capable of this role.

Yet good feelings, loving feelings about the person who is dying can lead the carer to fear the future. Anticipating your loss is very frightening. For couples who have been locked in a dependent relationship for years the loss will be all the more frightening. Fear about your future is a selfish fear and yet it is founded on your love. You are facing a loss that you will carry with you for the rest of your life. Although most people survive, and indeed find joy and contentment again, they face a time of dark depression. In the depths of bereavement life can seem not worth living, empty, a shadowland. Yet time and again I have seen patients hold on, waiting for the darkness to lift and eventually it does. Life takes on colour again. I recall a mother talking about the death of her son and even years later she said, 'but there isn't a day goes by that I don't think of him.' You will never lose your feelings but you will survive and you will be happy again.

Who is going to help you in your bereavement? Friends and family are most important. Professionals who have cared for you before the death can continue to look after you. Your GP or the hospice services can offer regular support, showing that they care and are still there to listen to you. Priest, social worker and voluntary carer may all be helpful too. As a GP I often see carers on a regular basis throughout these difficult times and I am glad to do it. Sometimes patients need a professional to ask the unaskable questions about how hopeless they feel. Some carers need treatment for their ensuing depression if they get 'stuck' in their bereavement. If you feel after a year that you can see no light at the end of the tunnel make sure you talk to someone about it. CRUSE is a voluntary organization that offers support to the bereaved. Their address is in your local phone book. The National Association of Bereavement Services will be able to put you in touch with a local group appropriate to your needs (see p. 238).

Angry feelings

You will probably have bad feelings: of anger, impatience and irritability. I expect even Mother Teresa got that way. So be assured that anger with your loved one is normal. Imagine how it feels to have a partner with lung cancer when you have nagged for years about giving up smoking. Perhaps you are angry that you had no choice in whether or not you became a carer. Or it may be the usual, more mundane anger we all feel when we are looking after someone—'If he rings that bell once more when I am trying to watch the news I shall go mad.' Simple routines may help you avoid battling or grouching with your loved one and then feeling guilty on top of everything else. Stop before you enter the patient's room, take a deep breath and count to ten, then try to go in with a smile. If you can't, and from time to time you won't be able to, analyse why you are so angry. Is it constantly being at the beck and call of someone or is it more complicated? Perhaps you can talk about it together. Can you come to some satisfactory arrangement where you have some protected time?

There may be anger with a selfish patient. One woman caring for a friend who was always discharging himself from hospital said, 'I used to lie in bed at night dreading hearing his footsteps on the stairs.' Several years later she is still full of anger about the way he treated her, the unreasonable demands he made.

Anger can also be an expression of the helplessness carers feel in the face of a relentless illness. Carers often feel angry with the loved one for not trying to eat, or not trying to help themselves.

Selfish feelings

It is quite common for carers to feel all attention is focused on the patient, and to think 'what about me—I'm suffering and need some help too.' This is absolutely true. For not only do patients develop unpleasant symptoms, the majority of their carers do too. Sleep problems, loss of weight, feeling nervous and anxious are all common and most carers suffer from one or more of these symptoms. You have to look after yourself if you are to continue to care effectively and that may mean seeking help for yourself. Your GP will see you and can prescribe sleeping tablets, but will probably do more good by listening and hearing your distress. Massage, relaxation techniques, yoga, all may have a role to play in caring for the carer. Acknowledge your own needs, and don't feel you are being 'selfish' in wanting care and concern shown to you too.

Exhaustion is a universal experience for those caring for a dying person, and of course nothing frays the temper so much as exhaustion. It can so undermine your strength that you can see no release possible until it is all over. There must be many carers who feel 'I can't go on, I wish it was all over and he would die', yet these are the kind of thoughts that most people will not share readily, perceived as truly 'bad feelings'. In fact they are very common and often shared by your loved one and his doctors and nurses as well as yourself. On several occasions patients have quietly asked me 'How much longer?' as they draw near the end. They too are weary and exhausted by the dying process. When I answer 'Not long now' a look of great relief comes over them. A GP recently said to me 'When a terminally ill patient dies it is both a sadness and a relief' and I identified with that. The waiting and the hard work is over but the sadness remains.

Waiting for the end is particularly difficult if you are expecting it sooner than it comes. The patient who is given three months to live and is still there at six months can foil even the best laid plans. In all difficult things we pace ourselves and a protracted death can feel rather like running a marathon in which the finishing tape keeps being moved back. Ordinary life is on hold and it is natural sometimes to long for its return at whatever price.

Anxiety

Anxiety crops up again and again when talking to carers. There are many possible focuses for it. You may be anxious about the demands of the present. Can you manage? The answer to that is you probably can, but you may have to define clearly what you mean by managing. A friend of mine recently talked about the death of her father. He had nursed his wife through her final illness at home, but when it came to his turn his loving daughter was clear that she 'couldn't manage the nursing, I can't bear those kind of things.' She grimaced at the thought. So he went into a good nursing home and she visited him every afternoon for the last two months of his life. With tears in her eyes she turned away from me, still sad after many years. Although she did not manage to nurse him she nevertheless showed that she cared for him by visiting regularly as clockwork every afternoon. If you cannot manage the nursing say so from the outset and make alternative plans. Perhaps you can undertake some of the care but there are some things that you just can't do. For example, dealing with a colostomy is for some people too difficult. Wiping the bottom of your loved one takes steadfast resolve and a certain gritting of teeth on both of your parts. You may have done it for your children but most of us never contemplate doing such things for our parents, spouses or friends. A surprising number of people do manage it, and understandably, a substantial number don't. If you fall into the latter camp, try not to feel guilty about it.

Anxiety about illness and death frequently manifests itself in a carer's inability to leave their loved one alone in the house. Statistics show that many carers stop going out and dedicate twenty-four hours a day to their caring role, sometimes for years on end.

Case history

The Underwoods are a charming old couple. When I visited recently they were sitting facing each other across their little sitting room, the gas fire on even in June. He has lung cancer and his breathing is getting difficult so that now he has trouble climbing stairs and is thinking of getting his bed moved down. He has been like this for over a year. His wife said she did go out round the corner to do the shopping 'and people stop me and ask how Harold is, but you know I put my head down and try not to stop and talk because I have to get back.' She likes to get back so that she can sit in the

> chair opposite and keep her eye on him. It is not
> rational, but her desire to be by him is so great that she
> cannot even stop for five minutes to chat with her
> neighbours.

If you are afraid to go out and leave your loved one
alone it might help to sit down together and list the
bad things that might happen if you did. Are they
rational or irrational? Show them to a third party
who may help you look at them more objectively.
Mr Reed, whose wife was bedbound for seven
years, had time away by using the Crossroads scheme
(see p. 225 for more details) which provided someone to sit with his wife twice a week. He got two
hours off and she enjoyed the company. Every six
weeks she went for one week of respite care at the
local hospital.

Perhaps you feel indispensable, that no one else
will be able to look after your loved one properly.
Again this is unlikely to be a feeling based on a
realistic assessment of the situation. No carer is
indispensable, and I do not believe that any carer
should dedicate twenty-four hours of every day to
that role. The Carers National Association (see
p. 224), a nationwide support organization, is very
helpful on these kinds of issues.

There may be considerable unspoken anxiety about
facing the moment of death, when suddenly your
loved one has gone and you are alone with their body.
For some people this is very frightening to contemplate, especially if they are likely to be alone in the
house. Perhaps you have never seen or touched someone after they have died. Many people have a fear of
body fluids erupting or staring eyes. You need not be
afraid of your loved one after death for nothing

frightening happens. The one alarming thing if you are not expecting it is that sometimes there is a slight gurgling or sighing noise of air escaping from the throat or a sudden shifting of a limb as muscles relax.

You will know when your loved one has died simply by the cessation of breathing. I always sit quietly at the bedside for a few minutes after the last breath has been taken, for occasionally with the Cheyne–Stokes breathing that precedes death there can be a long gap between breaths. There is an indefinable quality about the living person that disappears, and you will feel its absence. It is a moment full of mystery, not at all frightening if you are prepared for it. There is a profound quietness and calmness, and it is unlike any other moment you will ever experience.

It may help to plan for this moment in advance so that you do not feel panicky. Think about whether there will be other people there with you and, if so, whether you want to be alone with your loved one for a while or if you would prefer everyone to gather round to say goodbye together. You may want to hold your loved one in your arms again, kiss them goodbye. Perhaps you would like to make your loved one look comfortable, straighten their night-clothes or put on clean ones, fold their arms, shut their eyes if they are open, shut their mouth, brush their hair. It is up to you.

Who do you need to contact first? A member of your family or a friend may help by passing the news on to certain important people so that you do not have to make more telephone calls than necessary. Your district nurse may have left you her telephone number with instructions to ring her. You need to ring your GP or the deputizing service if she uses one at night, because at some stage she has to come and officially confirm the death. Having seen and examined your loved one she can fill in a death certificate giving the cause of death. She will also tell you what else you need to do. Ring the undertaker when you are ready.

The undertaker will come and lay the body out for you if you like, and they can either remove it then or leave it with you for as long as you like until the funeral. Perhaps you will be reassured by talking to the undertaker beforehand and discussing all these matters with him. Carers have said to me that it is important not to be rushed. If you want some time alone, say so. There is no hurry, no need for the undertaker to rush. Your loved one can stay at home until you are ready to let go.

Some people really do not want to see the body of their loved one and that is fine. The current orthodoxy is that saying goodbye by witnessing the body helps the grieving process. But it is entirely up to you and you must be guided by your own feelings. Talk to your district nurse about what to do immediately after the death and she can reassure you that there is nothing frightening or difficult. The nurses I work with give the sound advice of having a list of the telephone numbers you need by the phone so that everything is prepared. It does make things much easier.

At this stage a few people wish to do things differently. Some people may choose to make a coffin, or arrange the funeral without an undertaker dictating normal practice, and indeed such things may have been agreed previously with your partner. This is a new and powerful way of protecting your own autonomy but it can be fraught with difficulties because of the considerable suspicion of anything non-conformist. If you want to consider other options (you can, for example, be buried without a coffin in your own field), you should read *The New Natural Death Handbook* by Nicholas Albery which gives a clear account of all the possible alternatives.

Practical concerns

There are many practical problems that you will face as a carer and there are simple solutions for some of these problems. Perhaps you feel stretched to breaking point by trying to be nurse, housewife, breadwinner and parent all at once. 'I felt fully stretched before this and now I feel overwhelmed', said one of my patients recently.

What can you do to protect yourself and make sure that you continue to function effectively? Remember that your loved one will not be best served by an exhausted, fraught carer. You need to prioritize, organize, delegate.

Prioritize

What is most important to you, to your loved one and to your family? Is work and the financial security it brings essential to the well-being of your family? Perhaps it is the only thing that keeps you going, a necessary escape to the old, familiar and normal world. On the other hand, by claiming all the appropriate allowances and grants you may be able to survive without your income, and your stress levels might then fall.

Housework can be the straw that breaks the camel's back. For those who run an efficient, tidy house, keeping up your usual standards can be particularly difficult.

Many carers have children to look after, some deeply affected by the imminent death, others much less so. When an elderly relative is being cared for in a house with young children it may be difficult to accept that the children's schooling and social life should suffer. How are you going to strike a balance between what is best for the children and for the patient? Remember that children are resilient; some exposure to illness will not harm them, particularly where it is taking place in the safe and secure environment of home. Having children at home is not necessarily a reason to opt for hospital care. Children reaffirm the cycle of life, and bring some hope for the future into many sad houses.

Most carers complain that having to play hostess adds considerably to their burden. If you find yourself endlessly making tea, stop. Welcome your visitors warmly but do not feel compelled to do more work on their behalf.

Ensuring that you get some protected time away from your caring role might be another priority.

Organize

Organize your life so that you make some space for yourself. The longer your caring role is likely to last the more important this becomes. Family are usually very good at spreading the load, and many carers book a regular night off when they can go out of the house and have time just for themselves. Some hospices have a compulsory visitors' night off because they recognize how important it is for carers to have a complete break on a regular basis. Of course they make exceptions for relatives of the very sick.

Day and night sitters are a tremendously valuable resource. They give carers a chance to go out or have an undisturbed night's sleep, and they bring a fresh face into the house which is often cheering for the patient. Family and friends usually provide this respite, but the voluntary sector offers services to different patients. Crossroads, for example, will provide a sitter during the day or evening for young patients. Your church may have a volunteer who will sit in for you. Day centres and luncheon clubs provide many patients with a regular outing, and also give the carer a day off, and transport is provided which accommodates wheelchairs.

Night sitters are hard to come by and are mainly available for people with cancer. You may have access to Marie Curie nurses, specialist nurses who will sit overnight with patients (discussed further on pp. 57–58). Use them if you can, for they are wonderful. Some people do not want a stranger in the house all night and resist asking for such help, but once a family has started using the Marie Curie service I have rarely heard them express anything other than relief at the rest it affords them. Alternatively, a private nurse can be employed, but at considerable cost—currently in the region of £90 a night.

Respite care is a system whereby patients are looked after for a short time in a hospital or other institution specifically so that their carer can have a break. For some this is arranged on a regular basis; one of my patients with multiple sclerosis went into hospital, or a special wing of the local hospice, for one week out of six. Her husband cared for her at home for the other five. I must say she complained about it quite a lot, the food, the noise, the heat, but she recognized that it was a lifeline for her husband. For others a two-week respite may allow a family to get a much-needed holiday. Social services usually organize respite care so if you want to discuss this contact their local office. Alternatively ask your GP, district nurse or home care nurse as they will know what is available.

Nursing duties can tax the most robust carer. Generally, however, nursing tasks creep up on you, giving you time to learn or get used to one before the next becomes necessary. Ask your district nurse to give you some guidelines if you are unsure about anything. Particularly useful are simple rules about turning and lifting patients. The nurse can teach you and you can then teach your other helpers. Bed bathing and changing the bed are laborious tasks that can be approached in a methodical manner and made easier. See how your nurse prepares her tray with everything she needs to hand. Copy her and save yourself wasted minutes toing and froing to get things you have forgotten. The same is true for wound dressing; get a nurse to teach you properly so that you can cope with confidence. A little time spent at the beginning learning about these tasks will not be wasted. The Marie Curie Foundation has a simple instruction sheet for carers that you may find useful.

A ward sister has an important role in protecting her patient from too many or unwanted visitors. Ward routines also mean that most visitors can stay only for a relatively short time. Many carers find that they become the gate keeper, and this is a very difficult task. Insensitive visitors stay beyond the endurance of the patient, and families trying to maintain some kind of normal life may find that they are always entertaining guests. When people are trying to show that they care, it is a heartless task to have to turn them away. If this is a problem try to emulate sister and keep visitors to times that suit you and your family. Keep a rest time in the afternoon, and try to have an evening closing time. Some patients and carers find these simple rules easier to impose if they are sanc-tioned by the doctor or nurse: 'I'm sorry but the doctor has said no visitors after eight o'clock', or 'Nurse insists he must lie quietly after his midday medication and not be disturbed for two hours.'

Delegate

In these exceptional circumstances you should feel free to ask for help. Don't let friends get away with a breezy 'just let me know if there is anything that I can do'. Say 'Well, I do need someone to collect my pension every Thursday, perhaps you could do that for me.' If they say no, what have you lost? It is they who have lost face. Friends and neighbours will often welcome being able to do something really useful to help—after all, that is what a community is all about.

School children often need lifts to and from school, and need to get out to play as usual, to go on trips or to after school classes. Generally people rally round and help. School can be supportive too, if you talk to teachers and let them know your needs.

I can remember one carer who complained bitterly about all the visitors who came and never helped. On my next visit she had a mischievous glint in her eye. Upstairs I could hear the drone of the vacuum cleaner, while in the sick room her husband was being shaved by a neighbour. She had simply dele-gated some tasks to her regular visitors, and felt a great deal better for doing so.

Common Symptoms and Their Treatment

This chapter will give a guide to the common symptoms experienced in terminal illness and outline the current mainstays of treatment. Most patients will suffer from one or more distressing symptoms and some are very common—anxiety, sleeplessness and depression, for example. Others, like bed sores and constipation, can often be prevented if certain precautions are taken. The symptoms relevant to most patients and carers are considered first, and then further common symptoms will be discussed. Use them for reference. My aim is both to give practical advice that will help you recognize and manage the conditions yourself, and to look at the medical treatment currently available.

The symptoms are discussed in the following order: anxiety, p. 160; sleeplessness, p. 163; depression, p. 166; constipation, p. 167; Bed sores/pressure sores, p. 171; mouth care, p. 174; pain, p. 175; nausea and vomiting, p. 185; loss of appetite, p. 188; difficulty breathing, p. 190; loss of bladder control, p. 194; loss of bowel control, p. 197; confusion, p. 198.

Talking about your symptoms

Your symptoms are very important. They are not just an indication of your disease but of your disease.

They are not always easy to talk about. For the classic British stoic, of whom I number myself one, this seems to be particularly difficult. We often feel more comfortable denying our distress. Talking about difficult symptoms can feel undignified.

Yet you do need to describe how you are feeling, for research shows how bad doctors are at guessing patients' symptoms. Often patients believe their doctor will intuitively know how they are feeling. But doctors and nurses are not mind readers. You need to tell the doctor or nurse about your symptoms if you want them treated. Perhaps writing them down at the end of each day might help, for example 'Felt short of breath for ten minutes after having a bath this morning. Dull pain in my right knee all day. Worrying about my next hospital appointment a lot.' When the district nurse or GP next visits, the diary will serve as a check list so that you don't forget anything important.

Relatives often describe a patient's symptoms for them. This is very helpful, but it is still best to hear it from the patient. If you do feel more comfortable letting someone else speak for you that is fine, but perhaps you could explain this to the doctor making it clear that you consent to the discussion that follows.

Sometimes the carer reports a symptom that the patient denies: 'Every time I move him he winces with pain' is followed by 'No I don't' from the patient. Is the patient in pain and denying it, or is the carer projecting her own distress? Perhaps patient and carer are wrestling for control of the illness? To make a full assessment of the situation will take time, patience and tolerance, from everyone involved.

Occasionally patients need to keep their symptoms to themselves and do not want any treatment.

One woman with widespread cancer said 'I need to experience the pain.' It was real and it was hers. It is up to you what you do about your symptoms. Sometimes patients do not want to burden their family or their doctor with yet more problems. Your doctor is there to listen to you and help if she can. You will not be a burden.

What influences our symptoms?

Physical, emotional, social and spiritual matters all combine to influence the way we experience our symptoms. Physical pain can be treated with drugs, but this may not reduce the emotional pain, the fear, the anger, the depression, that accompanies it. Similarly, the symptoms of an illness will have social implications; becoming debilitated may lead to the loss of status at work or within the family, social isolation, or financial worries. Each person also has a spiritual self, some indefinable place within that can also be in distress. Everyone will have their own feeling about what that spiritual centre may be. When you are facing death it is natural to search for a meaning to your own life, to acknowledge fulfil-ment as well as failure and lost opportunities. It is also a time to look beyond the bounds of everyday life and find something greater to give meaning to your existence. The struggle to find a solution to the apparent meaninglessness of life is for many people the most painful journey that they have to make. By facing this trial and working through it, many are able to achieve acceptance of both life and death, and find spiritual peace.

If you get stuck wrestling with apparently unsolv-able troubles, you may find that it helps to talk about them. Some talk to family or friends, to a priest or to their doctor or nurse. Others find relief from talking to people who are less closely involved. Patients in hospital often find fellow patients are the ones who really understand. If you are at home you might be surprised to find who the 'right' person is for you. A young niece in her late teens recently turned out to be the listener that helped one of my dying patients. Everyone was surprised, because she seemed so young and inexperienced. Who knows what she brought to the relationship? The important thing was that by talking with her my patient was able to resolve something that allowed him to find peace.

Anxiety

I think it is true to say that anxiety is a universal experience for both patients and carers. It may fluctuate with peaks and troughs alternating frequently throughout the day. Everyone would expect you to feel anxious when you think about very frightening and difficult things, questions such as 'What will dying be like?' and 'What comes after I have died?' I hope that this book will go some way towards answering the first of these questions. Some people have their own answer to the second, but for many it remains part of the mystery that lies ahead and can be very frightening. Fear of the unknown is part of the human condition.

Obviously the future welfare of children, spouses or elderly dependants is likely to be foremost in many people's minds and the source of unremitting, sometimes overwhelming anxiety. These weighty matters may never be made all right but you can still take action to minimize the difficulty and hardship for those you leave behind. Sorting out your affairs as thoroughly as possible is helpful. Simply acknowledging your worries and doing something, however small, however inadequate, may ease the burden of your anxiety.

Sometimes anxiety keeps people hopelessly fighting death and prevents them from reaching a peaceful time of acceptance. A wonderful priest gives this example of how some people need to be 'given permission to die'.

Case history

A friend had cancer of the colon. She was the wife of a priest friend and I had been her spiritual director and confessor for many years. She had major surgery followed by radiotherapy and then had a very good year. Then there was a recurrence of pain with further surgery. She was a nurse and knew what her chances were. The doctors were openly honest and in spite of everything she opted for some very stressful chemotherapy. She struggled on at home for a few more months after this but things were getting progressively worse. There was a big haemorrhage and she was readmitted to hospital. My friend rang me thinking it was the end. When I went to see her she was in battling mood again and determined to get back home to do things again. I said to her, 'Who are you fighting for? Your husband and children all know what the score is. You cannot go on carrying them and they do not want you to go on torturing yourself. You love each other so much you have to face this reality together. The love you have for each other in the love of God is great enough to carry you through.' There was silence for a couple of minutes and then she said, 'You are right, it was for them but I don't know how much longer I could have gone on. Help me to give myself into the hands of God.' We prayed together and later that day her husband rang me to say a wonderful change had come over his wife—she was so peaceful now and they were simply going to live each day as it came and bask in their love and that of God for them.

Having been given, as it were, permission to die she lived for a further three months and the household radiated love to all who came to it. In particular she had an incredible effect upon all who ministered to her. Doctors and nurses and all who had visited her wrote to tell us so.

But it may not be these weighty questions that cause your greatest anxiety, something illustrated by this quote from a patient's recent thank you letter to the Cancer Relief Macmillan Fund. He was responding to a cheque they sent to assist him with his phone and electricity bills. 'Surprisingly, I was far more worried about my financial situation [getting the phone and electricity cut off] than the prospect of having only a few months to live.' Perhaps you are worried about your dog or cat and what will happen to them after you can no longer look after them. This may seem relatively unimportant to some people, but not to you. Just as a cheque for a telephone bill was the most effective way of alleviating one man's anxiety, so other relatively easy solutions may be available for yours. If you can tell someone your worries they may be able to help you solve them.

Sometimes though you may have a terrible feeling of freefloating, unfocused anxiety that can take hold of you, grip you and paralyse you. Probably everyone has experienced this awful feeling, but during a terminal illness it can come to stay. Talking may help, especially if you have a sympathetic listener who allows the waves of anxiety to wash over her, until eventually, perhaps, they seem to flow away. For others talk only leads round in ever tightening, tense circles and no relief can be gained that way. Perhaps a different way can be found to work with your anxiety and fear. Although not available on the NHS many find that massage or aromatherapy are most soothing and relaxing, and you may find talking easier once the tension has been unlocked. If you cannot afford a trained therapist ask your carer or a friend to wash and massage your feet, your hands or your back. It may be surprisingly therapeutic.

Occasionally anxiety becomes so overwhelming that medical treatment is needed, at least for a short time. Sedatives and anxiolytics, as they are called, can dull the edges and perhaps give you a breathing space. They are prescribed with caution because people become dependent if they are taken for too long. The new antidepressants can also be helpful.

Finally anxiety, particularly in the elderly, may be masking an underlying depression. Talking, and the tolerance born of understanding, may be the solution, but a concurrent antidepressant drug might also help.

Sleeplessness

A lot of patients have difficulty sleeping. The first thing to try to find out is what is happening to the sleep pattern. Is pain waking you at night? Perhaps you wake in the early hours and can't get back to sleep again— a sign of depression. Anxiety and fear stop you getting off to sleep and then keep waking you up. I think everyone knows the misery of lying awake in the small hours with the rest of the house sleeping peacefully. It can be the most lonely and frightening of times. Pain, depression, anxiety all need talking about and treating if possible. Occasionally the drugs you have been prescribed keep you awake. Dexamethasone is a particular culprit and if you are taking this twice a day try to take the second dose no later than lunch-time. Here are some simple guidelines that may help if you find that you are having trouble sleeping.

Try to aim for a quiet, restful evening, perhaps restricting visitors after eight o'clock. Take your evening medication remembering that sleeping tablets take twenty minutes to work. A tot of brandy or whisky might become a relaxing and comfortable part of your evening routine. Finally, settle yourself with a warm milky drink. Remember caffeine in tea and coffee can cause wakefulness so avoid these in the evening.

Keep the temperature warm and comfortable in the bedroom but open a window for fresh air during the night.

Then turn your attention to the bed itself. Is your mattress comfortable? Have you the right number of pillows for sleeping? Some people make a 'sausage' for the foot of the bed; this is a pillow wrapped lengthways in a sheet like a cracker, with the ends of the sheet tucked in under the mattress. This holds the bedclothes off the feet, which some patients find comfortable. It also stops you slipping down in bed during the night, which helps if you have difficulty breathing.

Even if you spend the day in bed it is worth marking night-time by smoothing out the bottom sheet, plumping up and turning over the pillows, and straightening the night clothes for a last time.

In the day try not to catnap. If you do need to sleep set aside a regular time—no visitors between lunch and three o'clock, say, so that patient and carer can take a siesta. Carers need to rest too.

Taking a little exercise is good. Even sitting in the garden getting some fresh air for a short time every day improves the quality of your sleep.

Perhaps you and your partner have always slept together in a double bed and now because of your illness you find yourself alone in a single. There is nothing better than a hug in the night to settle anxiety and let you sleep. Your district nurse may be able to supply a pressure mattress that can be fitted to a double bed.

If your pet has been a regular companion at night in your bedroom, don't banish him just because you are ill. One of the good things about being at home and not in hospital is that these parts of your normal life are not lost.

Sleeping tablets are very useful if you are not sleeping well. Even people who would never have contemplated taking them before find them effective. The type of sleeping tablet prescribed will depend on your sleep pattern. Some, like temazepam, get you off to sleep but their effect wears off in four hours. Others, such as nitrazepam, keep you asleep for eight hours, although some people find they wake with a slight hangover. Your doctor will choose the right type for you. If you need help with sleeping try one and see. You can use it from time to time, all the time, or stop it all together. It is up to you.

If you are waking in the night with pain, tell your doctor. She can change your painkillers to cover the whole night. If you wake early in the morning and can't get back to sleep your doctor may suggest trying an antidepressant. If your anxiety is overwhelming the best approach may be to treat this first, and a normal sleep pattern will follow.

Finally, don't worry about not sleeping. The worry keeps you awake, you sleep less, you worry more. In these circumstances have a plan up your sleeve. Think, 'blow this, I'm going to do something else'. Listen to the radio or a talking book (headphones will allow your partner to sleep), or get up and do a jigsaw or write a letter. Do something to break the cycle of worry and sleeplessness.

Depression

In Chapter 4 I described depression as one of the natural responses to a terminal illness, one of the 'stages' you will probably encounter as you come to terms with what is happening to you. Illness, particularly a final illness, seems to be defined by a series of losses: loss of independence, loss of work, loss of social life and sex life, each alone being enough to plunge anyone into depression. Grieving for those losses will take time, and it must be done.

There are, however, those who do get 'stuck' in their depression, and without help will not emerge from it. They often respond well to a combination of counselling and treatment with antidepressant tablets. If your depression is not lifting within three months it is worth asking your GP for help. The symptoms that are particularly indicative of a persistent and treatable depression are:

- low mood, and loss of interest and pleasure;
- tearfulness;
- feelings of worthlessness and guilt;
- belief that the future holds nothing worth living for;
- persistent suicidal thoughts or wishes;
- agitation, especially in the elderly.

Counselling can be given by your GP in short regular sessions if she feels confident to undertake it.

Sometimes you will need more time, and then some form of psychotherapy is needed. Recently, various brief psychotherapies have been developed which may be very helpful in this context. Your GP will be able to refer you to a local psychiatrist or psychotherapist or counsellor if you want. Antidepressant drugs are a standard treatment for depression, and do not interfere with concurrent psychotherapeutic treatment. They work by altering the level of certain natural chemicals in the brain that have become low in depressed people. They need time to build up in the brain before their effect is felt and this can take from two to six weeks. Keep taking the antidepressants, even if they do not seem to be working at first as they will in due course.

Some antidepressants help patients who are also experiencing anxiety and agitation. Your doctor will choose the one that suits you.

Some antidepressants have side effects which can be troublesome, particularly dry mouth, constipation and difficulty passing water. Most side effects settle to some extent over the first few days but you may have to weigh the benefit of the drug over the unpleasantness of the side effect. Of course this is particularly difficult when you don't feel the benefit for several weeks.

Constipation

The GP who trained me in general practice maintained that there were four things that people found particularly distressing: loss of appetite, loss of sex drive, loss of the ability to sleep and loss of a regular bowel function. When our bodies stop functioning normally there is an emotional component to our distress which often exceeds the discomfort of the condition itself. With constipation this is certainly true. But severe constipation is more than just distressing; it can have a profound effect on our bodies, and when severe can cause nausea, vomiting, abdominal pain, confusion and general debility. The doctor's aim is to prevent constipation ever reaching this stage.

Constipation is difficult to talk about. From early childhood we consider going to the lavatory to be private, and this silence is reflected in the impoverished language we have available to describe bowel function. If you don't know where to start just tell your doctor or nurse that you are constipated and let them give you their language. For example, if you told me that you were constipated I might reply, 'When you say constipated do you mean that you are opening your bowels less often than before, or do you mean that your motion has become hard?' I have given you words that I am happy using and you can use them back.

Opening your bowels anything from three times a day to three times a week is considered normal. Constipation occurs when you are going less often than is usual for you. There is usually an accompanying change in the consistency of your faeces which can become very hard and painful to pass.

It is common to become constipated when you are very ill for a variety of reasons. Often there is a change in diet and this affects the bowel. If less fibre is taken the faeces will tend to become smaller and harder. It may be possible to maintain a diet reasonably high in fibre, and this is certainly worth thinking about. You might try pieces of fruit as finger food, particularly dried prunes or apricots. Have a portion of fruit with every meal. Try wholemeal bread rather than white and perhaps a cereal containing bran such as Bran Flakes, Weetabix or Shredded Wheat each morning. Don't be too rigid about this, however, and above all do not force yourself to eat an unpalatable high-fibre diet. These are just suggestions that may help, they are not rules to be obeyed.

Drinking is very important as any degree of dehydration will tend to make you constipated. Regular small sips of any drink will help. Some people recommend a glass of water (warm if possible) three times a day. Others recommend a long fruit cocktail with or without alcohol before meals. The alcohol has the added advantage of stimulating the appetite a little, and many hospices have a 'happy hour' before supper for this very reason. If sitting up to drink is an effort try a cup with a straw or even a child's drinking cup.

When you are ill you need to rest and unfortunately we know that inactivity predisposes you to constipation. If you spend your day in bed you will probably become constipated. I think it helps to understand that your bowels are responding normally to their situation. They are not going wrong as well. If you can manage it, a little exercise will help, even if it is only walking around the house.

Some drugs have the side effect of making you constipated. Indeed, doctors know that everyone taking morphine should concurrently take a laxative. Make sure you do. There is now an alternative strong painkiller that I prescribe for patients who find morphine too constipating. It is called fentanyl and is given via a patch, like a plaster that you stick on your skin. The fentanyl is very effective at controlling pain without causing so much constipation, and the patch only needs changing once every three days.

Co-proxamol and other related drugs can also con-
stipate, as can diuretics, some antidepressants, iron
tablets, hyoscine and many others. You do not need
to take a laxative routinely with these drugs but be
ready to mention any change in your bowels to your
doctor. Prompt treatment can avoid the need for
enemas and suppositories later.

There are a number of laxatives available. Some
act to soften the faeces, others stimulate the bowel to
contract and move its contents through more
quickly. Your doctor or nurse will advise you on
which to take and you may need both types together.

If the rectum gets blocked with faeces, as sometimes happens when constipation goes untreated,
your district nurse can give a small suppository or
enema, or you can do this yourself. Ask her to tell
you exactly what she is going to do and what will
happen. A suppository is small and bullet-shaped,
like thick Vaseline. The nurse gently pushes it
through your anus into your rectum where it dis-
solves and softens the blockage so that you can get
your bowels moving again. An enema is used in a
similar way but it is a liquid squirted in through a
little plastic tube.

This all sounds awful, painful and undignified, but
in fact it is not necessarily so bad. Your nurse will be
neither disgusted nor embarrassed by the procedure
for it is part of her normal work. Try not to feel too
embarrassed yourself.

Some people are constipated because of an
obstruction in the bowel, and these patients will
receive their initial treatment from a specialist. I
would just like to mention the existence of specialist
stoma nurses for those who have had a colostomy or
iliostomy. They are expert in teaching you how to
cope with the physical problems that may ensue.

Emotionally it can be very difficult for the patient, and sometimes for the carer, to adapt to life after a colostomy. You may both need to talk about these feelings with each other and perhaps with the nurse. The address of the British Colostomy Association is listed on p. 224 and you may find it helpful to contact them.

Bed sores

Bed sores are also known as pressure sores and that is just what they are. Pressure sore is a better name because they are just as likely to develop sitting in a chair as lying in bed. They occur where the blood supply to an area of skin is reduced because of pressure, and they can develop in a matter of hours if the pressure is not relieved. The affected area of skin dies, exposing the tissues below. The sores can vary from the size of a five pence piece to several inches across, and they are often painful. They are a miserable thing for any patient to have.

When you are ill and weak you become more prone to developing pressure sores, for several reasons. You may be much less mobile so that you bear your weight on the same areas for long periods. If you have become thin you may take most of your weight on bony prominences, such as the heels, buttocks, lower spine, elbows and shoulder blades. Even the ears can be affected. Because the weight is not evenly distributed over the body, the pressure on these areas is vastly increased. Poor nutrition and sometimes the process of the disease itself both make your natural ability to heal less efficient.

Preventing pressure sores takes a lot of work but it pays off handsomely. Once a sore has developed it can take weeks to heal, and the pain can be difficult to control. If you consider the way in which pressure sores are caused you will see the rationale behind the various preventive measures. Here are some guidelines for their prevention.

The first is to keep moving, changing position before the skin of one area can become damaged. If you are sitting in a chair, try to get up and move around for a minute every half an hour or so. If you are lying in bed change position regularly. Nursing the very weak or unconscious patient in bed is a formidable task for the carer. A counsel of perfection is to turn them from one side to the other every three hours, day and night. Ask your nurse for advice about this, as she can teach you how to move the patient without hurting your own back. She may also be able to provide you with aids like a slide sheet that help you to move the patient more easily. A pillow wedged behind the patient's back will stop him rolling back. Another between his knees will stop sores developing where the bones lie on top of each other and rub together.

There are many other ways of relieving pressure on bony areas, but these should be used as well as, not instead of, the above measures. Sheepskin is a wonderfully versatile material which can be used in booties to protect the heels, as a chair seat for the buttocks, or as a mattress. Spenco cushions or mattresses are an alternative and may be provided from district nursing stores. Foam heel protectors called Tubipads are available on prescription. A piece of foam to support the back when sitting in a chair may help, especially if you cut a hole where the lower spine rests so that there is no pressure in that area.

In bed attention should be given to the bottom sheet. Make sure it is not all wrinkled up. Bed clothes should be light and a 'cradle' can be put under the foot of the bed to hold the covers off the feet. If your nurse cannot supply one, a cardboard box can be cut to shape and used instead, but check with your nurse before using it as rough edges may catch the skin.

Each day as the patient is being washed and dried the skin should be inspected for sore areas. Again, your nurse will show you where to look and what to look for. Aqueous cream can be rubbed into any vulnerable area of skin. It is inexpensive and can either be prescribed or bought from your chemist. Areas of redness that take a while to fade are a sign that the skin there is in danger of breaking down. Look out for shiny skin or small breaks. Some nurses protect all the very vulnerable areas, and certainly those that are looking red and shiny, with a 'second skin' called Tegaderm. It looks like clingfilm and can be left on for several days.

The most difficult problem arises when the patient has become incontinent, for wet sheets rubbing against the delicate skin soon cause it to become sore. Incontinence pads may be available through the district nurse. A draw sheet or baby cot sheet with a plastic sheet underneath make changing a wet bed quicker and easier. Sometimes it becomes necessary to catheterize a patient (run a tube from the bladder out via the penis or urethra into a bag). Although as a patient you may think this sounds awful it is not too uncomfortable once you get used to it and, as ever, it is a matter of balancing the advantages over the disadvantages. Certainly if your carer is having to turn you every few hours a day and night plus change a wet bed in-between times, it may make a difference between them coping or becoming too exhausted to carry on.

My mother is a doctor, and she maintains that in her day no patient in hospital ever got a pressure sore; matron would have taken it as a personal insult if you even suggested such a thing could happen on her ward. These days things are different, and sadly patients are sometimes discharged home with pressure sores that have developed while in hospital. So although the thrust of this section has been on prevention, I think carers struggling to do their best for their loved one must understand that the task can be formidable even for a team of nurses in hospital. If you have done your best and still a pressure sore develops, do not reproach yourself. However conscientious you are they still sometimes appear.

Once a pressure sore has developed the district nurse will come and dress it regularly but it can take a long time to heal. Of course it is still important to continue with your preventive measures.

Mouth care

Our mouths are usually moist and quite clean, without us paying them much attention. In illness this can change for a variety of reasons. Less saliva may be produced, often as a side effect of the drugs being given. It is also more common to breathe through the mouth, which will make it dry. If you are weak and eating and drinking little you can become dehydrated, which leads to a dry mouth. Weight loss may cause dentures to stop fitting and this can cause problems with dribbling and soreness at the corners the mouth. Regular dental appointments tend to be abandoned with the onset of serious illness. Find out if there is a community dentist in your area who can, if necessary, visit you at home. Another common cause of soreness is oral candidiasis (or thrush) which appears as flecks of white—like milk curds—on the inside of the cheeks of tongue. Ask your GP or district nurse to check as it is easily treated.

The most effective way of keeping the mouth clean is to brush regularly with a soft toothbrush, using water or toothpaste. If you become too weak to do this let you carer take over, brushing twice a day as part of a general washing routine.

If the mouth is dry, research has shown the best treatment is to use a replacement synthetic saliva spray which can be prescribed for you. Try it and see if it makes you more comfortable. Alternatives are regular mouth rinses, and I think that water is as good as anything, although nurses generally favour adding a little bicarbonate or other cleanser. Sucking boiled sweets, slivers of ice on the tongue, or cubes of frozen juice are all comforting. Crushed pineapple is particularly good as it contains a natural enzyme that helps clean the mouth.

Dry lips can be eased by regularly applying Vaseline, glycerine or lipsalve. Vaseline does not taste too good, and some say glycerine dries the mouth further. Try them and see which suits you. If you become very weak your carer will need to be shown how to clean around the inside of the mouth and tongue. A soft toothbrush may still be the most effective way of doing this. Alternatively the nurse will provide plastic forceps and gauze swabs and show how to clean the mouth gently. Attention to small details like these makes all the difference.

Pain

Pain is perhaps the most feared of all symptoms. Nearly three-quarters of people suffer some pain when they are dying, yet almost everyone can have their physical pain relieved with drugs. The aim of treatment is to make a patient completely free of pain for twenty-four hours a day, though sometimes this will have to be accomplished more gradually than you as a patient might wish. You and your doctor may aim first for you to be completely pain free at night, then when at rest during the day, and finally free of pain even when you are moving.

Acute pain occurs in response to tissue damage and we can anticipate it getting better as the body heals. Chronic pain, on the other hand, arises from damage where healing is not anticipated, and this is the commonest cause of pain in terminal illness. It is also the pain of diseases such as arthritis. More than one type of pain can be experienced at any one time.

Patients use their own language to describe the pain they feel: 'like a knife twisting in my side', 'like a sore tooth', 'worse than being in labour', or as a Bangladeshi patient said to me, 'Doctor, I have too much pain.' These descriptions bring the pain to life and help the carers empathize with the patient's distress, which is a good start. Your doctor or nurse needs to know exactly where the pain is and how long it has lasted. Excellent control is achieved by thinking very carefully and precisely about your pain. Does it come and go or is it constant? How does it affect you? Does it stop you doing anything? Does it wake you at night? Each time treatment is started or changed they need to review all these aspects of the pain. An experienced doctor or nurse will be able to discover the answers to these questions during the course of a normal visit. She will generally ask all of these questions while she is talking to, or examining, a patient. She will also observe the patient carefully, as body language and facial expression communicate as much as words do. The stoic who says 'I'm feeling fine, doctor' but winces when gently moved is obviously in pain and needs to be encouraged to describe his symptoms. Similarly, it is hard to misinterpret the drawn and unhappy look of a patient with chronic pain, nor the change that comes over her when that pain is banished.

It is well documented that patients find pain more intolerable if they are anxious, frightened, depressed or unhappy. In terminal illness you are often beset by all these feelings. Your doctor should be prepared to treat you with drugs that are strong enough to banish your pain. However, you may be able to reduce the amount of drug needed by reducing your level of distress. Talking about your feelings often eases them. Relaxation aided by massage, meditation or yoga may reduce tension and anxiety. Complementary therapies that treat your depleted energy state may also be very helpful.

If you can analyse how you feel about your pain, understand what it signifies and allow yourself to acknowledge how frightening it can be, you may find that you feel more in control of it.

Drug treatment

There are now simple guidelines for the management of pain in terminal illness, particularly in patients with cancer.

Doctors start with a 'ladder' of painkillers: weaker drugs are at the bottom and get progressively stronger on the way up. The aim is to match the drug to the pain so that you take the weakest drug that will give you total pain control. If the pain gets worse you go up the ladder until you are free of pain again. Your doctor will decide where you should start. Sometimes if the pain is severe a strong drug is needed straight away. A good GP or district nurse will assess this and will start you at the right level.

Some types of pain, however, do not respond to this regime and they are treated differently (see p. 184). As they are less common I am going to concentrate on the usual approach to treatment. Here is a summary of the ladder:

- *Step one*: regular aspirin or paracetamol.
- *Step two*: regular weak opioid, such as co-proxamol, DF-II8, co-codamol 30/500.
- *Step three*: oral morphine at the dose needed to control the pain.

It is very simple. Suppose your GP starts you on paracetamol and the pain goes. That may be all you ever need. However, if after some weeks the pain returns, you stop the paracetamol and go up a step. The next group of drugs are the 'weak opioids' so your GP prescribes co-proxamol regularly every six hours, and again the pain goes. If it returns while you are on this regime, you will stop the co-proxamol and go up a step. The point is that you and your doctor do not waste time trying the other weak opioids, shuffling around on the same step trying the other drugs 'in case they work'. You must get rid of your pain, because pain grinds you down, makes you irritable and miserable, gets in the way of life. If you are still in pain your GP will then prescribe morphine.

The 'morphine myth'

Morphine is an excellent painkiller and has become the mainstay of treatment for intractable terminal pain. But patients usually feel ambivalent about starting morphine and you too may feel this way.

For many people the step up to morphine feels like admitting defeat, as if they are now starting the final journey. It is not surprising that suffering some pain seems preferable to this. I understand this feeling. Yet I often find myself trying to persuade patients that they would, in fact, be better off taking morphine. I know that some patients need morphine for a while but then their pain eases and they can then take a step down the ladder. Needing morphine does not mean you are giving up the fight against your disease. The fight against your disease is a fight for life. Patients fight better for their life when they are out of pain.

People associate morphine with dying and worry that it will kill them. Recently a patient of mine steadfastly refused to take morphine. Two years earlier she had nursed her husband at home when he was dying of lung cancer. In the end he became very breathless and was admitted to hospital. The doctors started him on morphine and he died within twenty-four hours. My patient believed the morphine had killed her husband though he was admitted to hospital because he was dying. Morphine sometimes appears to kill patients if it is started right at the end. Better to use it as soon as you need it and reap the benefit of its power.

One of the common side effects of morphine is drowsiness and this deters some patients. When the drug is started or the dose increased there may be an initial period of drowsiness but this should pass; if it does not, the dose of drug can be adjusted. Sometimes patients chose to experience some pain rather than be drowsy.

Both patients and carers often express the fear that morphine will lead to loss of control and to addiction. In fact when morphine is used to treat pain it seems that its addictive properties are utilized fighting the pain so patients do not become addicted. If the pain subsides there is rarely a problem reducing or stopping the drug. Morphine does, however, affect control, especially when it is first started and the patient is drowsy; it is as if consciousness is clouded. One woman I know described how she felt that her mother had 'gone' once she started morphine, 'for the last three days of her life she was not really there.' Probably this was as much the disease as the drug. Many patients live ordinary day-to-day lives on very high doses of morphine and remain very much themselves.

Finally, patients understandably fear that they want to save morphine for later when they 'might really need it'. Be assured that your doctor or nurse will not offer you morphine unless they judge that you really need it now. Your body will not get used to it; it will not stop working.

Morphine and all the other opioid drugs work by binding to receptor sites on cell membranes which are mainly found in the brain and spinal cord. Think of the receptor sites as a lock and morphine as a key. By turning the key in the lock your experience of pain is turned off. Morphine needs to be taken regularly over a period of time to get maximum effect. This is because it is metabolized or changed by the liver into slightly different forms. The one form that is particularly effective at turning off pain takes a while to penetrate into the brain and unlock its receptors.

Side effects

But the opioid receptors don't only turn off pain. They also unlock some other doors and this is why they have side effects. As with all drugs the wanted effects have to be balanced against the unwanted ones. These are the common side effects:

Nausea and vomiting: nearly one in three patients will experience nausea and vomiting when they first start morphine or when they increase the dose. It settles after about five days and during that time will need treating with an antisickness drug and haloperidol is the one that is usually used.

Constipation: all patients on regular morphine will become constipated and so need to take a regular laxative.

Dry mouth: this is another common side effect which needs treating with regular mouth care, such as rinsing or freshening with mouth swabs.

Drowsiness and confusion: about twenty per cent of patients feel drowsy for a few days after starting or increasing the dose of morphine. Once the dose is stabilized the symptom will subside within two to three days. If a patient remains very sleepy the dose of morphine will need reducing.

How to take it

Morphine can be given as a liquid, a tablet, a suppository or by injection. Usually doctors start with a small dose of liquid which needs to be taken regularly every four hours. The idea behind giving it every four hours is so that your morphine receptors remain permanently unlocked. Do not wait for the pain to come back before you take it. Another reason for starting with four-hourly medicine is that it is then easier to make small adjustments to the dose. Tell your doctor or nurse if you are still experiencing pain, because now is the time to establish very good control. You can either increase the quantity of medicine you take every four hours, or the strength of the medicine. At this point you would not change the length of time between doses.

If, however, pain 'breaks through', rather than wait for the next visit by your doctor or nurse, your carer can give you an extra dose of morphine. Your nurse will explain exactly what to do. She will ask you to write down the dose, the time and what the patient was doing when the pain occurred. The next day she can readjust the regular dose appropriately to stop the pain breaking through again. This sounds more difficult than it is, and you will soon get the hang of it.

Once the dose of morphine you need has been established, your doctor will change you on to special tablets which have the great advantage of being taken only twice a day. They release the drug slowly over the course of twelve hours and are called morphine sulphate continuous, MST or Zomorph.

There is no maximum dose of morphine, your doctor will prescribe as much as you need. Don't worry that you are taking a lot. Some people need hundreds of milligrams a day and they can still be up and about, getting on with their daily life.

Regular review

When you are stabilized, your doctor or nurse will want to review your situation on a regular basis. They will need to know about side effects; constipation, for instance, should be routinely treated.

Are you remaining free of pain or has some returned? If breakthrough pain becomes frequent it is sometimes necessary to go back to four-hourly medicine in order to work out exactly what dose of MST is needed. This is dispiriting, but worth it in the long run. Sometimes other drugs will be used as well. Ask your doctor or nurse to explain what they are giving you and why. If you understand the rationale behind your treatment you are much more likely to feel happy about taking it.

Injections

If you are vomiting or having difficulty swallowing, if you are extremely weak or have slipped into a coma, oral medication will have to be stopped.

Usually the drug is then given via a needle either as a regular injection or continuously under the skin. In recent years a small machine called a syringe driver has revolutionized terminal care by allowing drugs to be injected very slowly over twenty-four hours, providing a constant level of the drug to circulate in the body, with minimal inconvenience to the patient. The machine is small and light and you can easily carry it around. Once a day your district nurse will fill a syringe with the drugs you need and clip this into the syringe driver, which is battery operated. Then via a thin plastic tube that goes under your clothes the drugs slowly pass to a tiny needle. The nurse will slip this under the skin of your upper arm or body and secure it with a plaster. Once in place most patients seem to forget about it. If the area gets sore the needle is moved, but often it can stay in the same site for several days at a stretch.

Morphine is not very soluble so a similar drug called diamorphine is used in the syringe driver. Other drugs for sickness can be added if necessary.

Many, but not all, GPs and district nurses have their own syringe drivers or have access to them from the local hospital or hospice. The syringe driver has an alarm which will sound if there is a problem. This is actually very rare. Whoever sets up the syringe driver will leave you a telephone number to call in case this happens, and the nurse or doctor will come round and sort it out. In reality it is much less alarming than it might sound, and after the first few days patients feel quite at home with their syringe driver.

Pain requiring special treatment

In nine patients out of ten morphine provides good pain control. A few patients do not get relief while others find that the side effects are intolerable even with the correct treatment. In these cases a different strong drug from the opioid group may be tried. There are a number to choose from and the one we are now using most frequently is called fentanyl (Durogesic). This is also an opioid but it unlocks a slightly different group of receptors so that although it is effective at controlling pain it is significantly less constipating than morphine. What is interesting is the way the drug is 'delivered' to your bloodstream. It comes in patches, like rather large plasters, that are stuck on the skin of the upper arm or body. The lovely thing about them is that they only need to be changed every three days. The first patch takes twenty-four hours to work properly so extra pain relief may be needed initially. The dose can then be adjusted every seventy-two hours when the strength of patch can be changed as necessary. Patients can safely change their own patches. There are a number of other strong painkillers that can be tried if patients have other intolerable side effects or for the few who have what is known as 'morphine-resistant' pain. If you are running into these kind of problems, or if after a short time it is clear that your pain is not coming under control, I think you should see a specialist.

Many district hospitals run pain clinics for patients with difficult pain problems. Hospice doctors, who are particularly skilled at managing intractable pain, can either do a home visit or you could go to the hospice. Sometimes it is necessary to admit a patient for a few days in order to control their pain. Seeing you throughout the day helps the doctors and nurses understand the pattern and intensity of your pain, and plan appropriate treatment.

Certain types of pain respond better to other specific treatments. In these cases your doctor may not follow the rules of the pain ladder. Pain from cancer in the bones, headache from raised pressure in the brain, liver pain, nerve pain or muscle spasm all need special consideration. Your GP may initiate this treatment at home, or you will need to see a specialist. The best treatment for the pain of a cancer secondary in the bone is radiotherapy, for example. One single treatment may be enough, but it means a trip to the hospital.

Not all hospital doctors are specialists in pain control and most hospital consultants are no more skilled than GPs. So when I say a specialist I do not necessarily mean your surgeon, or regular hospital consultant. Your GP may refer you to an anaesthetist, a palliative care specialist, a radiotherapist or hospice doctor depending on the type of pain you have.

Nausea and vomiting

Feeling sick is rather like being in pain, in that it gets in the way of life. Add to this the distress caused by vomiting and you have a truly miserable situation. You fear going out in case you vomit, and mealtimes, which are usually a sociable and enjoyable part of everyday life, become just another duty to be got through.

Unfortunately it is a common symptom and one that can be difficult to treat effectively. In deciding on the best treatment your doctor must first identify the cause of the problem; she will need to consider whether the symptoms arise from your underlying condition, or whether they are a side effect of the drugs you are taking (like morphine). Constipation, infection, indigestion and even anxiety can cause or exacerbate the symptoms. Your doctor has to take time to think about these various causes, and she will probably want to examine you too. Once a diagnosis is made she can choose the most appropriate drug for you.

Antisickness drugs are given by mouth or absorbed through the skin (often a drug-impregnated patch is put behind the ear). Alternatively the drug can be given in liquid form via a syringe driver through a tiny needle under the skin (see the description of a syringe driver on pp. 183–4).

Rather like painkillers, antisickness drugs should be taken regularly throughout the day, and you should not wait for your symptoms to return before taking the next dose. Take the first dose when you wake but don't get up for half an hour as walking around seems to make nausea worse and lying still relieves it. After half an hour the medication will have started working and you can get up and try some breakfast.

Some patients find that the drugs make them drowsy and then you are faced with trying to decide where the best path lies between symptom and side effect. As a patient you get the last word on this and professionals and carers must respect your decision not to take treatment if that is what you want.

As well as tablets there are some other helpful things you can try. First think about reducing your exposure to the smell of food as there is nothing worse when you are nauseated than to have cooking odours wafting around. Obviously cooking has to go on in the house, but the kitchen door should be shut. Keep a window open and an extractor fan on if you have one.

Spicy and aromatic foods may be particularly unwelcome as may the smell of greasy fried food; some of these smells will be inevitable, but be aware of the problem.

When I was pregnant I was tormented with nausea and vomiting for several months and found that certain perfumes and cigarette smoke made me feel awful. If this is true for you, explain to the offending person. They can easily change their perfume next visit, or go outside to smoke.

It is hard to know what to eat when you feel sick. As a general rule small tasty meals are preferable, and moist food is often easier to swallow. One of the nurses I work with swears by salmon sandwiches— small, tasty, healthy and moist, just rather expensive on a regular basis. But if you are not eating much else perhaps the expense is acceptable. Another suggestion is to suck a piece of lime to freshen your mouth and then have a little of what you fancy. In season, a buffet of cold cuts and salad will allow you to join in a sociable meal with family or friends and not feel exposed if you only choose to eat a little.

Consommé or Bovril drinks can be nourishing and are as good as a meal. Fizzy drinks are often better than tea or coffee at settling the stomach. Sucking ice cubes seems to help some people.

If you are vomiting regularly have a bowl by your chair or bed. Knowing it is there is reassuring and reducing the anxiety associated with any symptom is always worthwhile. After vomiting you may like to rinse your mouth, so always have a glass of water to hand.

If vomiting is persistent in spite of treatment you may need to be seen by a specialist from a hospice, and perhaps admitted in order to try to bring it under control. Sometimes the improvement is miraculous and starts the moment you step over the threshold. Clearly if this is the case there is a psychological component to your symptoms which responds to the inherent safety of the hospice environment. Exploring your anxieties about being at home may be the mainstay of treatment.

Loss of appetite

This common symptom is very distressing. We take pleasure in eating every day of our lives without really giving it much thought. It is not until our appetite goes that we realize how we miss it.

In cancer and AIDS a loss of appetite and weight loss are often part of the disease process. The loss of weight is not directly caused by lack of nourishment and so cannot be reversed by feeding with high-protein foods. It is very hard to believe that you cannot feed a patient up and give him strength to combat his disease but nevertheless it is true.

Carers are often more disturbed by the loss of appetite than is the patient for it seems to signify the inexorable progress of the disease. How can he get better, get stronger if he doesn't eat? I remember an elderly Jewish patient weeping because her dying husband would not drink her chicken soup—chicken soup, known also as 'Jewish penicillin' because of the faith many of her generation put in its nourishing, healing properties. He could not eat it, he was too ill, and she felt impotent as a result. I think that this is the underlying emotion that informs all our other responses to a loss of appetite. Carers need their distress to be heard, and should feel free to talk to their doctor or nurse about how they feel.

There are things that can be done and the first is to exclude a treatable cause. Loss of appetite can be the first sign of impending nausea, so it is worth trying an antisickness drug. Constipation, infection and depression are other treatable causes. A sore mouth is relatively common in terminally ill patients. Any infection in the mouth, particularly candidiasis (which looks like white milk curds), can be easily treated. Loose-fitting dentures can cause soreness and some drugs make the mouth dry.

Once treatable causes have been excluded you will probably want to adapt eating patterns to suit the new situation. It is very dispiriting to sit down to a large plate of food and then to fail to eat it. So try a little attractively presented food on a small plate. Finger food beside your chair or bed allows you to snack intermittently. In general savoury food is often more palatable than sweet, cold rather than hot and moist rather than dry.

If you are looking after an elderly patient remember that they may be at home with a more old-fashioned diet than you are used to. An experienced nurse who now runs a residential home for the elderly suggests you offer a little steamed white fish in white sauce, which is moist and tasty. Custards are similarly comforting and nutritious. Towards the end, when very little is being taken a spoonful of fruit yoghurt or a little ice-cream are both easy to swallow and pleasant.

Some patients find it easy to take liquid food supplements, and your district nurse will be able to recommend the different flavours and types. It can be very comforting to know that although a patient is not eating he is getting some balanced nourishment in this way. They are by no means necessary but try them if you feel like it.

Appetite stimulants do exist and are sometimes used, although this is a controversial area. There is no disagreement about alcohol though—an aperitif will stimulate the appetite which is why a 'happy hour' is part of the daily routine of many hospices. Drugs are generally used only when weight loss is a particular cause of psychological distress. The side effects of the drugs must be balanced with the bene-fits to the patient. Sadly, eating more and gaining weight due to drugs will not slow the progress of your disease, but for some patients it alleviates distress and is therefore beneficial.

Carers must try never to pressurize the patient into eating. Keep meals small; your body will tell you what you need and remember a little of what you fancy does you good. And there is still pleasure to be had in giving and receiving food. I will never forget visiting an elderly patient of mine in a small council flat in Hackney. Mrs Freedman was totally bedbound and unable to speak following a series of strokes. Mr Freedman was sitting on the side of the bed feed-ing her strawberries. He turned and said, 'Every June we like to treat ourselves to a few strawberries, don't we, Lil?' and the smile on her face answered yes.

Difficulty breathing

Anxiety and fear

We breathe without thinking, and to find breath-ing difficult is extremely frightening. When we are anxious we naturally breath faster. This panic breath-ing makes our breathing feel even more difficult and thus we enter a vicious cycle. Sometimes it is necessary to treat the anxiety in order to break the cycle.

Patients with breathing trouble sometimes have a horror of choking to death. I remember one man who was so overwhelmed with this fear that he had completely withdrawn into himself. I admitted him to a hospice where, surrounded by doctors, nurses and technology, he felt safe. His fear subsided, and he was able to die peacefully ten days later. In fact patients hardly ever choke to death and you need not fear this. The natural mechanism of the body allows you to fall into unconsciousness as your breathing deteriorates. Sufferers of motor neuron disease are often very fearful of choking, yet new research from Exeter University has shown that nearly all motor neuron patients die peacefully. The Motor Neurone Disease Association has a truly excellent leaflet called 'How will I die?' which I fully recommend (see p. 234 for address).

Treatment

Treatment for breathlessness varies according to its cause. For example, if your breathlessness is due to heart failure you will receive completely different treatment from someone with a pleural effusion or fibrosis of the lung. You can ask your doctor to explain the rationale behind your treatment. In hospital, breathless patients are often given oxygen and this is also available at home, delivered in a metal cylinder that can be placed by the chair or bed. You breathe the oxygen through a face mask attached to the cylinder by a tube. Oxygen is not a panacea, however, and many patients will not benefit from having it at home. Some find it reassuring to have a cylinder in the house in case they need it. Others are dependent on oxygen for many years. Oxygen is available on prescription, and your chemist will deliver it regularly to your house.

Some drugs can be given via a nebulizer which is a machine the size of a briefcase that can be used both in hospital and at home. Either your GP or hospital specialist can initiate this treatment. Drugs are vaporized by the machine and breathed in through a face mask. Each treatment lasts about twenty minutes. Nebulizers are sometimes available on loan but often patients buy their own from the manufacturers; currently the approximate cost is £120. Knowing that treatment is always at hand helps allay the anxiety associated with breathlessness.

A small dose of morphine can ease the sensation of breathlessness. If you are already on morphine for pain your doctor may increase the dose by fifty per cent to help your breathlessness, but if you are not on it a small dose every four hours may be effective. Diazepam, more commonly known as Valium, can also be used if you are feeling very anxious, as can the cannabinoid nabilone.

All patients with compromised breathing will be vulnerable to chest infections. If the infection is caused by a virus, for example the influenza virus, antibiotics will not help. But for bacterial infections they are standard treatment. Unfortunately some antibiotics can only be given by injection. If you need antibiotics injected you will almost certainly be admitted to hospital for at least a few days.

In very sick patients who are near to death pneumonia is often the final event, and is sometimes referred to as the 'old man's friend'. It may be kinder not to treat rather than leave the patient with even more severe breathlessness for the few remaining days of life. This is not euthanasia; it is about having the courage to recognize that there is nothing further to be gained by postponing death. Patient, doctor and carers all need to be involved in making the decision, and it is at times like this that you need a family doctor or nurse that you can really trust.

Self-help

If you are having difficulty breathing you will generally be more comfortable in an upright position or even leaning slightly forward. Pillows placed on a table or bed table in front of you will allow you to rest comfortably forward on your arms. You can buy a back rest or a special A-shaped pillow which gives good support when sitting up in a comfortable arm chair or in bed. A 'sausage' made by wrapping a pillow lengthways in a sheet and tucking this under the sides of the mattress at the foot of the bed helps prevent slipping down.

Loose, open-necked clothing should be worn, and fresh air may also help, so have a window open or a fan to circulate air in the room. Sufficient humidity is also necessary. Visitors should try not to sit too close to the patient. Simple physiotherapy can help drain secretions in the lungs. If those caring for you have not been taught how to do this by a physiotherapist in hospital, your district nurse will be able to show them. If you are very sick, however, you may find this too exhausting and so it is inappropriate. When a lot of sputum is being produced containers need to be near at hand, and small empty margarine tubs with a lid are as good as anything. Your local chest clinic may be able to provide further specialist advice if you need it.

Cheyne–Stokes breathing

In the last hours as a patient is dying his breathing often becomes laboured and irregular. This is called Cheyne–Stokes breathing. Although it is distressing to witness, the dying patient has usually lapsed into a coma, and is certainly not troubled by his symptoms. Nurses and carers can sit with him keeping him comfortable, but he has no need of treatment. The noise of saliva rattling in the throat can be very upsetting for carers. Repositioning the patient can sometimes help and if the noise is very distressing there are drugs we can give to reduce the secretions that cause it. The one person who is not distressed by the noise is the patient himself and sometimes when carers realize this they find it less unbearable themselves. I think doctors are treating the carers' distress at this point, and it is kinder to leave the patient in peace.

Loss of bladder control

Most of us have not been incontinent since early childhood, and the loss of control implied by incontinence is very distressing. It was humiliating to wet the bed as a child and it is humiliating again now. With sympathetic treatment and time you may be able to adapt to your new situation. You may find ways of re-establishing control, not necessarily over your bladder, but over its effect on your life and your feelings.

A doctor will aim to treat any reversible cause and to minimize discomfort and inconvenience and the physical work of the carer.

A urinary infection can sometimes make a patient incontinent. The diagnosis is easily made by sending a sample of urine to the laboratory and treatment is an antibiotic for a few days. Other underlying causes should be considered; what drugs you are taking, for example, as some, particularly diuretics, can precipitate incontinence. Treatment of confusion or constipation may lead to an improvement in urinary symptoms.

If incontinence is an intermittent problem it is worth adapting your clothes. You can undo jogging pants much more easily and quickly than zips and buttons; they can be thrown in the wash and need no ironing. In the day they look as if you have got up and dressed, yet you can comfortably get into bed with them on as well.

If getting to the toilet is difficult, men can use a urinal, a special bottle that you can have by your chair or bed. It is designed to minimize spillage. Some men cannot pass water lying down, and they may prefer to move to the edge of the bed to use the bottle. I have always wished that there was an easy female equivalent but there isn't although a slipper bed pan is worth trying. Alternatively a commode can be provided by the nurse if you would like. Patients who are bedbound can usually be helped out onto a commode placed next to the bed.

There are a number of pads available, some for the bed, others that you wear. Ask your district nurse to tell you what there is as provision varies greatly from one district to another. In some areas there is a maximum limit on the number of incontinence pads a patient can have in one year so you may need to contribute towards the cost.

If you remain very wet even with pads, it may be more comfortable to use a bag. For men there is a bag attached by plastic tubing to a penile sheath which fits the penis like a condom. The bag can be strapped to the calf and you can walk around normally. Alternatively, both men and women can be catheterized. Your doctor or nurse gently pushes a plastic tube via the penis or urethra, into the bladder. A little balloon is inflated inside to stop it from falling out. The tube and bag arrangement are as described above. If you try a catheter it can easily be removed if you do not like it, but many patients get used to having one and it is lovely never to wake with a wet bed. Common problems that arise are bladder infections, which are easily treated, and blockages, which cause pain as urine fills the bladder and is unable to escape. Be assured that the bladder never bursts, but you will need a visit from your doctor or nurse straight away. They will either unblock the catheter, or remove it.

When a patient is bedbound their carer will need to devise a way of changing the sheets with minimal effort. A plastic mattress cover can be bought from any large department store. Try a cotton draw sheet with a waterproof back, on top of the normal full-sized sheet. The draw sheet can quite easily be changed.

Attention needs to be paid to skin that is getting wet regularly, as rashes can easily develop. Wash and dry the affected area twice a day and apply a barrier cream such as Conotrane cream, Vaseline or zinc and castor oil. Your GP or district nurse can prescribe one if necessary.

Another problem is smell, which can be very depressing, though it may in fact be far less noticeable than you imagine. A good system for bagging up used pads helps. Black bin bags are good for sheets awaiting washing or collection by the laundry service. Pads can be wrapped in newspaper then disposed of in plastic carrier bags which can be tightly tied and taken out to the bin straight away. There are electric air fresheners, sprays, perfumed oils or candles, provided they are acceptable to the patient who has to live in the room with them. An open window is cheaper and a jasmine in flower more beautiful to look at.

Ask your district nurse or social worker if any help is available to deal with the extra laundry. There is a laundry service for some patients. You may be able to get a grant to buy a washing or drying machine.

When you are at home incontinence can be a great trial for both you and your carer, and if this all gets too much you may eventually choose to go into hospital. If either of you feels this way do try to talk to your doctor or nurse before you reach crisis point. Together you may be able to find a way of coping with this most difficult of problems. Many districts have specialist incontinence nurses who can give you advice. They probably understand better than anyone how distressing incontinence can be.

Loss of bowel control

Loss of bowel control, or soiling, is less common than urinary incontinence but nevertheless occurs at some time in nearly one-quarter of dying patients. Many of the strategies suggested for urinary incontinence are equally applicable. If you develop this most distressing symptom you and your carer will both need support and understanding from all the professionals who are involved in your care. Your district nurse and GP will probably have several patients in the same situation as you. Don't feel that you are alone. Ask for their help and together it may be possible to develop your own method of coping that helps keep life tolerable in what initially appears to be an intolerable situation.

The commonest treatable cause is, paradoxically, constipation. The rectum becomes blocked with faeces and liquid builds up behind this blockage until it starts to seep around the sides. The patient appears to have frequent runny diarrhoea. With vigorous treatment for the constipation the incontinence should be resolved. If, however, your incontinence is due to diarrhoea your doctor can prescribe medicine to make the stool more solid. Sometimes a regime of antidiarrhoea medicine and regular enemas helps keep the rectum empty.

Confusion

It is tremendously frightening to imagine becoming confused, losing control and becoming entirely dependent on others. Yet for many the anticipation of mental deterioration is worse than the actuality. Most patients who become very confused are no longer frightened. For the few who become very distressed and disturbed there is treatment. Just as doctors would not hesitate to treat physical pain, neither would they leave a patient in mental torment. Occasionally this means sedating a patient so that he sleeps most of the time, rather than leave him distraught.

A degree of confusion is quite common when a patient is approaching death. Often this is due to a combination of dehydration, a rising level of urea in the bloodstream as the kidneys start to fail and the cumulative effect of the drugs that are being given.

The kindest thing at this stage is to reassure the patient gently that they will always be lovingly cared for and explain that their confusion is not a sign of madness but is part of their illness.

If confusion develops earlier in a terminal illness its cause must be thoroughly investigated because it is quite often reversible. Where it is not reversible it is equally important to have a clear diagnosis so that appropriate care can be planned. Elderly people, some of whom are already suffering from Alzheimer's or similar conditions, are most likely to suffer from confusion, while others are tipped from clear consciousness into a state of confusion by their illness.

Drugs are a common cause; any patient who suddenly becomes confused must have their drugs reviewed by their doctor. If one drug in particular is identified it can be stopped or changed—in most cases an alternative can be substituted. Next on the list of common causes is infection. Confusion may be the first sign of a chest or urinary infection and these are easily treated. Severe constipation can have the same effect, and sorting out the bowels cures the confusion. High levels of circulating calcium, common in bone cancer and myeloma, is another treatable cause. It can be diagnosed at home with a sample blood test.

Other causes are more difficult. For example, low levels of oxygen or high levels of carbon dioxide in the blood both lead to confusion. As these are usually due to chronic lung disease or severe heart failure all the available treatment is generally being given. Breathing oxygen may help a little and is worth a try. Brain tumours and secondary deposits that have spread to the brain from a cancer elsewhere can be treated initially with steroids. This may improve the confusion or delay its progress, but it cannot stop the inexorable progress of the disease. When this is the case it is very important for the patient to have the situation fully explained. Similarly, patients who are suffering multiple small strokes need to know they may become confused in the near future if the strokes continue; in order to continue to exert some control after the onset of confusion it is essential to have made arrangements beforehand. This is why it is important for the patient to understand as early as possible the implications of his disease. In Chapter 4 I discuss the legal steps you might wish to take to ensure that you will get the kind of continuing care you want.

For carers the onset of confusion in their loved one is desperately sad. It is also alarming and difficult to cope with. Having assessed the situation with the help of your doctor and made sure that any reversible cause is treated, you must decide whether or not you can continue to manage at home. Ask if there is any extra help available, a home help, or a night nurse, perhaps. Ensure your doctor or district nurse understands the problems you face.

If as a carer you feel overwhelmed by the onset of confusion in your loved one perhaps you will find that some of these suggestions for coping will help you. Confusion often ebbs and flows with resulting periods of complete clarity in which the patient understands exactly what is happening. These are the times to seize. Any important unfinished business should be dealt with as quickly as possible.

Patients often find that their long-term memory is much better preserved than their memory for recent events. Gently seek out these pockets of memory and then talk around them. Encourage family to talk about familiar things. Try to avoid chatting over a patient who is unable to follow the conversation or join in. Perhaps now is the time to stop well-meaning acquaintances and neighbours from visiting, as it is difficult for the patient if he cannot exactly place the face at the bedside. One old friend or family member at a time is easier than a group.

Try to avoid disagreeing or arguing with a confused patient, but help them by doing your best to inform them gently of their mistakes. For example, I visited a patient who thought I was her hairdresser. Rather than just put her straight I deferred to her mistake by saying 'Yes, I know I look very like her but actually I'm Dr Lee, your doctor.' Of course sometimes it may be difficult not to argue. A man who was looking after his confused father became increasingly angry every morning when he found that the old man had wet the bed. Finally one morning the son in exasperation said, 'Why have you wet the bed again?' The old man honestly did not think he had, and so replied, 'I didn't wet the bed', to which the son retorted, 'Well, who else could have, there wasn't anyone else in bed was there?' In his confusion and distress the old man just became more and more muddled, and the son immediately regretted his outburst. There is no right or wrong in this story, and every carer must at times lose their temper. I tell it to illustrate the point that you cannot argue rationally with someone who is confused.

When patients are very confused it may be impossible to understand the content of their talk, yet nevertheless you can sometimes understand the feelings they are expressing. This gives you the means by which you can communicate with them, and is like opening a door into their confused world. It enables you to say, 'You sound very worried about the things you are telling me', or 'How frightening that sounds, is that how you feel too?' Sometimes this can be a way of reaching a confused patient and helping to draw him back to your reality.

The great advantage of being at home is that the environment is familiar. Patients' confusion often becomes worse when they are admitted to hospital, which is not surprising if you consider the myriad of new stimuli that have to be noted and stored in the short-term memory. New faces, new noises, a new route to the toilet. It is the short-term memory that is most compromised in confusional states.

Adjustments can be made at home to make life easier for the confused patient. Recently I went to visit an old lady who was growing increasingly disorientated and confused. As part of my assessment of her mental state I had to ask her the date and the approximate time of day. Before answering she looked up at the clock and then surreptitiously glanced at the date on her newspaper. 'Four o'clock in the afternoon and it's the 4th of January 1994' was her correct reply. Later she told me that her mother was living around the corner and she was hoping to see her tomorrow. Her mother had been dead for thirty years, and she was in reality extremely confused. But she still knew how to use the prompts around her to help orientate herself. A good-sized clock in the patient's room, and something showing the date may be useful for all confused patients. An intercom or baby alarm can be useful as it will allow a carer to listen out for a confused patient from another room.

Doctors should have checked sight and hearing in elderly people as they can become very isolated when their senses are failing, which can precipitate confusion. A hearing aid, glasses or a magnifying glass can often improve the quality of their life immensely. Wandering patients are a great worry to carers, particularly when they get up at night. Falling out of bed is another problem. Some simple measures can minimize risks here: the district nurse may be able to provide a hospital bed with cot-sides for home, although a little imaginative positioning of furniture will do just as well. Armchairs pushed against the sides of the bed are quite effective. A toddler's stair-gate at the top and bottom of stairs reduce another potential danger.

Confusion can make feeding more difficult—a feeding cup can reduce spills. Similarly, getting to the toilet in time may become difficult, so having a urine bottle near at hand and trousers that are easy to get down may reduce accidents. Paying attention to small details like these is a very important way of maintaining the dignity of the confused patient.

Cannabis

Finally, it is worth considering the role that cannabis has to play in treating the symptoms of terminal illness. Although it remains illegal in the UK it is very widely used, both for recreational and therapeutic reasons. Cannabis is not a single drug but a complex mixture of chemicals. Indeed there are sixty cannabinoids present in raw cannabis. It has been shown to have an effect on a wide range of symptoms including pain, nausea and wasting in cancer and AIDS. At present the world's biggest clinical trial of the cannabis plant is being undertaken in Plymouth to look at the effect of cannabis oil on pain and tremors associated with multiple sclerosis. The research is particularly aimed at identifying the dose that will relieve symptoms with minimal side effects. Although people generally enjoy the cannabis high many patients do not want to be stoned when they have to take the drug all the time.

In March 2001 the House of Lords Select Committee on Science and Technology called for an end to the prosecution of genuine therapeutic users who posses or grow cannabis for their own use. In this prevailing climate I think it very unlikely that anyone would consider prosecuting a terminally ill patient for cannabis use.

If you smoke cannabis regularly you probably know a lot about the drug and what dose suits you. If you don't and you want to try it you should talk to an experienced user.

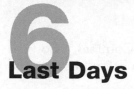

Last Days

This chapter of the book is about death itself. You may not feel ready to read it but it is here if you need it, and it can wait.

The time surrounding death is intensely personal and intimate. I have had the great privilege of listening to carers talk about the deaths of their loved ones. Sometimes the events they described felt too private for me to write about. Yet all those concerned have read this chapter and have agreed to share their stories in this way. Our hope is that those facing death may gain strength and courage from reading them. Some of the common experiences that precede death are recounted, followed by very moving descriptions of the moment of death. The chapter and the book ends with the carers' descriptions of letting go of their loved one to whatever lies ahead.

These are part of the stories of Bramwell Gould, a boy of ten who died after a year of illness, and of Keith Goodman, a young man who suffered from cancer of the spine. Both remained gracious, uncomplaining and loving to the end. Atilio Lopez, also young, fought against his death, ran from it, but at the very end came home in the most remarkable and defiant manner to die with his friends beside him. Here also are the stories of two elderly women,

Elizabeth Thomas and Louise Cornford, who both had time to say goodbye to life before slipping into unconsciousness and death.

Saying goodbye

As death approaches many patients prepare by finally putting their affairs in order and saying goodbye. Sometimes dying people seem to review the whole of their life as part of the process of saying farewell.

Louise Cornford was seventy-five when she died. People called her the 'hippy granny'. She first felt ill at the beginning of December and from that time her energy just seemed to go. Within four days she was in pain, which she chose not to have treated—it was as if she needed to experience it. Her daughter Alison sat with her and she talked and talked, about her childhood, her husband, her children—things her daughter had never heard before. After this she seemed to be retreating into her pain. Alison describes these days as 'so rich, so full, and yet there was a day to dayness about them. In the morning I would go home to the children, everyone would go to work. It was like a different world up in that flat. All those yesterdays coming in.'

Soon Alison's brother arrived and it was agreed to call the rest of the family while Louise was still conscious. Her sons came but her elder daughter, Jane, was on a yacht in the Virgin Islands and could not be contacted. Alison was given the job of trying to get a message to her but Louise said 'Don't call her.' The boys said goodbye to their mother and left saying 'You'll be better soon, we will see you soon.' Louise herself felt that she had said goodbye for the last time and was ready to die. But she didn't die. She woke up next morning in a furious mood and said 'Why am I still alive?'

On a Monday two weeks before she died Elizabeth Thomas made a will. The next day she sat down with her daughter-in-law and got out all her jewellery and decided exactly who should be given what, remembering her grandchildren, godchildren, daughters-in-law and sisters. She had one grandson with whom she sat and talked about the afterlife and her conviction that after death she would not be gone. Next she saw her vicar and planned her funeral down to the last detail, including the hymns and who should read the lessons—and who should not!

Her daughter-in-law, Lucy, sat with her one day and Mrs Thomas talked and talked about her whole life—her childhood, her sons and how proud she was of them, how glad to see them both settled, her marriage, her religion, her work. The following day her two sisters and their husbands came to tea. For the first time during her illness she did not get dressed. They talked about the past and watched old films of the children. That night she went to bed and never got up again.

Keith Goodman had been cared for by his mother and brother with a remarkable amount of help from Keith's friends, all young men and women in their twenties. They had sat with him through long evenings in hospital. When he came home they looked after him every evening between five and half past ten which allowed his mother to go upstairs and rest in preparation for the night when she sat by him. Up to twenty friends would be packed into the small front room night after night, laughing and joking with Keith. Sometimes they would take him out in his wheelchair to restaurants, clubs and to football matches. Then in May Keith said 'Mummy, I don't want to go out anymore. I'm too tired. I need time to sleep and think.'

By the end of May he was confined to bed. Gradually his speech became slurred and he could do nothing for himself. By the middle of June, when he could barely talk, he began to say goodbye. He said 'Hug me Mummy, squeeze me, this is the last time I am going to see you,' and he squeezed her to him as hard as he could. His mother was crying over his shoulder, but when she sat up and looked at him she put on a brave face.

Then Keith's close friends visited, and he asked them all to do little things for him—give him a sip of water through a straw, straighten his sheet, give him a kiss. It was his way of saying goodbye.

Distress

In the days or hours preceding death there is often a period during which people become very distressed. It usually occurs when they have stopped taking food and water and it may in part be due to dehydration. I think of it as a period of transition, just as in childbirth a labouring mother experiences a time of distress, panic and loss of control as labour reaches its climax and the baby is ready to be born. And then the distress ends. There follows a precious time of waiting, of anticipation, filled with either joy or sorrow.

Bram was only ten when he died. Throughout his year-long illness he was incredibly brave and uncomplaining. In the end he developed pneumonia. With the fever that accompanies pneumonia people often become confused and lose control and this happened to Bram for a few terrible hours. While he was distressed and frightened it was difficult to understand what he was saying. He seemed angry, pushing his mother away, saying 'Go away, Mum, you're absolutely useless', and later, 'Go away, why can't you make me feel better?' He pushed away water, oxygen, everything. His mother, Maryanne, describes feeling 'so helpless, so inadequate, awfully frightened.'

Their GP came and gave Bram a morphine injection. After this he became calm and peaceful.

Elizabeth Thomas became very distressed two nights before she died. She had stopped eating and drinking. Her daughter-in-law, Lucy, was sitting with her and she kept repeating 'Lucy, quick, quick' in an agitated way, as if Lucy should do something to comfort her, though nothing she tried helped. Her distress lasted all night. In the morning the district nurse arrived and catheterized her in case she was distressed by a full bladder. Later her GP came and after discussion with the family arranged to start a syringe driver with something to settle her. Shortly after she became calm and lucid again.

This period of distress is very common and very frightening for patient and carer. Often it passes naturally; if not, treatment can be given to speed its passing. It nearly always heralds a time of peacefulness, when the atmosphere in the sick room is one of calm. Nothing more needs to be done. It is a time of watching and waiting.

Last hours

The story of Atilio is included here because he did things differently. It illustrates that there are as many ways of facing death as there are individuals in this world.

Atilio had AIDS and had asked his communal household in London to look after him until he died and these five friends had agreed as a group to look after him when the time came. Sacha, with whom I talked, shared his care with Cora, Jamie, Steve and Sally, as well as having support from many others.

Just before Atilio died he came out of hospital, very weak and thin. To everyone's amazement and dismay he announced that he was going to Paris. No one knows how he did it, but he went. Cora and Sacha felt torn. Should they get on with their lives, or should they wait at home to see if Atilio would come back? They decided not to wait around.

Two days later a call came through to say that Atilio was coming home and needed collecting at Gatwick. Jamie went. He arrived to find the airport in a state of uproar. Atilio was lying on a stretcher, barely conscious. Jamie had no car, and so with help Atilio was lifted onto a train and then brought by taxi to their house in Great Russell Street. Everyone carried him upstairs to his beautiful attic room and he was gently laid on his bed. By now he was unconscious. Sacha and Cora had been called home and Cora arrived first. A doctor came and left after confirming that there was nothing more that anyone could do but wait. Then Sacha arrived. She was sure that Atilio knew she had come. The two women sat by him watching and waiting. Sacha did a drawing of him.

After half an hour the women turned to each other and said, 'God, it's cold.' They looked at Atilio. 'Do you think he's dead? Is he dead?' They held his hand, they held a mirror to see if he was still breathing. It was a fantastic moment; a relief that it was all over and that he was there with them, that he had made sure that he was there with them at the end.

The day before Elizabeth Thomas died a priest came
and sat with her, and she talked lucidly for the last
time. In the afternoon, shortly after he had left, she
slipped into unconsciousness. Her son's first wife sat
with her that last night. They no longer turned her
every three hours for she was clearly dying. They
didn't want to disturb her.

During her final day she was peaceful. Her breathing was laboured and there was a continuous rattle in
her chest, like snoring. Her husband came in and out
to see how she was but found it too distressing to sit
with her. Her young grandchildren came in and out.
Her son and daughter-in-law sat with her alternately.
At nine o'clock that night they turned her on her
side to reduce the rattling noise, and then they
encouraged her husband to come back in. Within
three minutes her breathing had become very shal-
low. 'I think she is going,' said her son, at which his
father let out a howl of pain and ran out of the room.
Lucy was torn between staying with her husband or
running to comfort her father-in-law, and chose the
latter. Elizabeth Thomas died with her son beside her
a few minutes later.

Keith Goodman opened his eyes for the last time on
June 22nd. Ten friends were there to say a final goodbye. For a week they had been expecting him to die
but he was so strong that he kept on going. At
10 p.m. the night sister came and together with his
mother she washed him and turned him. Then his
breathing became heavy and changed. His eyes were
clear but, as his mother said, 'he wasn't there'. His
mother and brother sat by him and his mother knew
death was close. She held his hand and called to him
and he shook but could not respond. At 1 a.m. his

brother could bear it no longer; he left the house and went to his girlfriend. Soon Keith broke out into a sweat. Mrs Goodman wiped his brow. At 3.10 a.m. he died and as he did so his body, contorted by spinal disease, readjusted in the bed. Within twenty minutes he had straightened up. His mother says 'It was a peace for me when I saw him die, his suffering had stopped. I didn't cry then, I was too pleased.'

When Louise Cornford eventually started taking morphine for her pain her daughter Alison felt that somehow she had gone. She moved in and out of consciousness. That night for the first time Alison did not want to sleep in the same room as her. 'I suppose I was afraid that she would die. I had come to terms with her dying but not with the actual fact of her death.' She slept nearby with the doors open between the rooms. That evening a party started in the flat upstairs, with thumping music coming through the ceiling. Louise just said, 'Oh, they are having a party,' and seemed unconcerned. Alison could not bear it and she rushed upstairs and said that her mother was very ill. When they realized how serious it was the neighbours immediately turned off the music and there were flowers on the doorstep the next morning.

And then her sister Jane arrived with Louise's granddaughter, Ems. A message had got through to them in the Virgin Islands. By now Louise had lost both sight and hearing. Jane put her hands on her mother and Louise said, 'That's Jane, isn't it? I knew you would come.'

Jane sat with her mother that night and at six in the morning she called Alison for there was a rattling noise in Louise's chest. Although she was unconscious, they sensed she was in pain so they called their GP who came straight away. Alison, Jane and Ems were all in the room. With great tenderness the doctor gave her a pain-killing injection, and she died almost at the same moment. Afterwards Alison describes feeling 'completely elated'. Jane said 'I want a GP like that.'

When Bram developed pneumonia his GP told Maryanne that he would probably die within twenty-four hours. He said it would be cruel to treat Bram and left saying 'We must make him as comfortable as we can. I'll go and organize help for you and get everything to you as soon as I can.' It took several hours for this to happen which seemed to Maryanne like an intolerable delay. During this period Bram seemed distressed. Maryanne called her ex-husband Phil, who was Bram's father, and he came. Their friend Gabrielle was also there helping in any way she could. The previous month they had gently said to Bram's brother, James, 'You know Bram's not going to make it, James' and when James came home from school that evening they told him that Bram was dying. He started to cry. Gabrielle was very close to James and she looked after him all that night. It was the only night that James did not sleep in the bedroom that he shared with Bram.

Their district nurse came and stayed until nine o'clock and then a Marie Curie nurse arrived. Bram was kept comfortable. He looked peaceful. Bram had been confined to bed for the previous month and all that time his cat and five kittens had never moved from his bed. Suddenly that evening they got up and left.

Bram's grandparents arrived. Phil and Maryanne sat at either side of Bram all night. At 4 a.m. he squeezed their hands for the last time. At 6 a.m. his breathing changed completely. A short time later he died, cradled in his parents' arms. At that moment Maryanne experienced 'a tangible feeling of love. Like giving birth. Agony and incredible love.'

Letting go

The moment of death passes. In that moment everything is profoundly changed. Yet the ceremony of care and love goes on, the carers performing their final physical acts of caring before they let go of the body they have loved and tended for so long.

Atilio's carers came together for the last time with him just after he had died. Everyone in the house came up to his room and sat round his bed with Sacha and Cora. They stayed there with him for a long time drinking and talking. They didn't lay his body out or move him or anything. 'We didn't know how to do any of those things,' Sacha said.

Keith's mother phoned her ex-husband as soon as their son had died. Together they put him in fresh pyjamas, combed his hair, closed his mouth. 'He looked so lovely, you could hardly believe it was the same person. His colouring came back and he looked as if he was in a beautiful sleep. He looked himself again.'

Elizabeth Thomas's son and daughter-in-law folded her hands and closed her mouth. When she looked nice they encouraged her husband to come back in and say goodbye.

After Bram died no one left the room for ten minutes. Then James came in. He put Bram's favourite teddy in bed with him and wept and wept. Then everyone silently left so that Maryanne could be alone with Bram. Later her friend Sue, the district nurse, came and together they laid him out. Maryanne was not ready for him to be taken from her so she asked James, 'Do you mind if Bram stays?' 'It's a bit weird, isn't it?' he replied, but he did not mind. Bram stayed in Maryanne's bed and she sat with him all day. She lit a candle next to him and friends came to say goodbye.

On the first day he was 'very much still around' for Maryanne but by the second he had gone. Then the undertakers came and took him next door into the church.

When Louise Cornford died her daughters went into the sitting room and opened a bottle of champagne. Then Alison went home to give a birthday present to her youngest daughter and take the children to school. Jane and Ems were with Louise for a while and then Alison came back. They had been advised to ring a local undertaker who said they could be there in half an hour. 'No,' she said, 'I need longer than that. I need two hours.' She did not know what she needed two hours for but she knew that she needed to be alone with her mother. 'I don't know how you would like me to send you off, Mummy,' she thought.

Alison felt that her mother's spirit had been trapped ever since the morphine started. She lit candles in the room. It was a beautiful, cold, crisp morning so she opened the windows wide. The white curtains billowed in the breeze and Alison felt her mother's spirit leave the room. She let her go.

Appendix 1: What to do After a Death

- You must contact your surgery to get a doctor to come and confirm the death. Usually your own doctor will be the one to come but if she is away or off duty whoever is covering for her patients will come instead. Once this done you can contact the funeral directors. When the surgery is next open your own doctor will give you the following:
  - a **medical certificate** certifying the cause of death (addressed to the local registrar);
  - a **formal notice** stating that the doctor has signed the medical certificate and telling you how to get the death registered (you must register a death in the area in which it has occurred).

- Occasionally a death must be reported to a coroner. In these cases the coroner will issue the death certificate. Where it has been an expected peaceful death at home your doctor will only report the death to the coroner if she did not see the deceased within fourteen days of the death, or if death was attributable to an 'industrial disease'.

- You can stay with your loved one for as long as you feel that you need to say goodbye. You need not feel rushed, you can contact the local funeral director and ask them to come when you are ready.

- You must act quickly if the patient wished to donate organs for transplant (normally these must be removed within half an hour of death so this may not be possible if the death has occurred at home). Consult your doctor. You can donate

corneas from the eyes for up to twenty-four hours
Contact your nearest eye hospital.

- If you have not discussed funeral arrangements
  and there are no instructions in the will, you
  should contact a funeral director for a written
  quote.
- You may want to consider a non-religious ceremony
  as an alternative to a funeral service, which can
  mark the passing of a human life with equal
  poignancy. The *New Natural Death Handbook* and
  the booklet *Funerals Without God*, published by the
  British Humanist Association, are good sources of
  information (see p. 241).
- For comprehensive details of the above plus all
  other issues arising at the time of a death I suggest
  you get leaflet D49 'What to do After a Death'
  from your local social security office.

Appendix 2: Checklist of Statutory Benefits

This list is a brief summary of benefits available as of 2001. For further information call the Benefits Enquiry Line 0800 882200.

Attendance allowance: this is a tax-free weekly cash benefit for people aged sixty-five or over who need help with personal care because of an illness or disability. It is paid to the patient to help pay for day or night care at home, but you can claim it even if no one is actually giving you the care you need. You can spend it any way you want. You must normally have needed care for six months before you can claim. If you are terminally ill this is obviously inappropriate and so there are special rules. Your doctor must sign a medical report stating that you are unlikely to live for more than six months (form DS 1500) and you or your carer can complete a claim form from your local social security office. Very few doctors are willing to predict how long a patient is likely to live, but they will all sign this form if you have a terminal illness, erring on the pessimistic side in order to get you the allowance. It is paid weekly and is currently £30.80 for people needing help by day or night, £53.55 for people who need help day and night—derisory when you consider that a private nurse will cost about £90 a night, but still worth claiming.

Disability living allowance: this is tax-free benefit for people who need help with personal care, with getting around, or both. It is for people under sixty-five. There are two components: a care component and a mobility component. Most people will not be able to claim until they have needed help for at least three months and are likely to need it for at least a further six. As with the attendance allowance, special provision can be made if you are terminally ill. You can be eligible for as little as £14.20 a week or as much as £90.95 depending on your disability.

Invalid care allowance: this is a weekly cash benefit for people aged between sixteen and sixty-five who are giving regular and substantial care to a severely disabled person. You must be spending at least thirty-five hours a week as a carer and be earning no more that £72 a week after deduction of allowable expenses. You currently get £41.75 for yourself. You may also get £24.95 for a husband or wife, or an adult who looks after your children, and about £10 for each child.

Home responsibilities protection: if you cannot work because you have to stay at home as a carer, you may be able to protect your right to the basic retirement pension or widow's benefits for your wife. It reduces the number of qualifying years you need for a full basic pension.

Other cash help: income support, family credit and the social fund may all provide people on low incomes with financial help. There is a cold weather payment and a funeral payment and community care grants can be given for all kinds of things, such as furniture, removal costs, minor house repairs. Social services can also provide grants for various things: a telephone, washing machine, holiday. If you have identified anything that would ease the burden of caring work contact them and see if they can help.

Free prescriptions: these are available to everyone over sixty-five years old. If you have a continuing physical disability, and terminal illness can count, you can get free prescriptions by filling in form FP91 available at your surgery or the post office.

Charities: they are a rich source of help and patients often feel overwhelmed by the generosity shown them in their time of need. It really feels as if someone cares. For patients with cancer the Cancer Relief Macmillan Fund (CRMF) provides one-off grants and so do many other organizations. They have simple rules: only patients currently with cancer or suffering from the effects of cancer qualify for a grant. They must not have capital in excess of £6000 for a single person, £8000 for a couple and their net weekly income must not exceed £100 per individual. There is a CRMF application form that needs to be filled out by a professional health or social worker. Most health and local authorities stock the form, if not ring the CRMF welfare officer, telephone number 0207 8407840. If you qualify for a grant, ask your doctor, nurse or social worker to help.

Here are the CRMF categories of need for which grants are awarded.

1. Clothing	2. Furnishings	3. Fuel	4. Holidays
clothing	bed	fuel	convalescence
footwear	bedding	heater	holiday
laundry	carpet		holiday fares
wig	chair		holiday
	cooker		insurance
	fridge		outings
	furnishings		
	liquidizer		

mattress
microwave
shower
tumble dryer
TV
vacuum
  cleaner
washer/
  dryer
washing
  machine

5. Miscellaneous	6. Care	7. Telephone	8. Travelling
bed and	child	phone	car insurance
breakfast	minder	extension	car mainte-
decorating	home	reconnection	nance
general debts	help		tax/licence
general	(six		visiting fares
expenses	weeks)		
kennel fees	home		
miscel-	nursing		
laneous	(two		
mortgage	weeks)		
arrears			
paper			
tissue			
prescriptions			
rates			
removal			
expenses			
rent arrears			
toiletries			
TV licensing			

Appendix 3: Useful Sources of Information and Support

General

Age Concern
Astral House, 1268 London Road,
London SW16 4ER
Tel: 0800 009966
Contact the head office for further details about local groups and publications.

Association to Aid Sexual and Personal
Relationships of People
with a Disability (SPOD)
286 Camden Road, London N7 OBJ
Tel: 020 7607 8851
SPOD provides an information, advisory and referral service for disabled clients, and also information and training for professional workers.

British Association for Counselling and
Psychotherapy (BACP)
1 Regent Place, Rugby, Warwickshire, CV21 2PJ
Tel: 0870 443 5252
Website: www.counselling.co.uk
BACP publishes lists of qualified psychotherapists and counsellors working in your area. Such lists may be held in a good reference library or are available free directly from BACP. Please send an A5 stamped addressed envelope stating your needs.

British Colostomy Association
15 Station Road, Reading, Berkshire RG1 1LG
Tel: 0800 328 4257
Provides support and advice for people living
with a colostomy. Run by area networks of
volunteers who themselves have colostomies.
They can arrange visits at home or in hospital
on request. Directory of local contacts available
on request.

Carers National Association
20–25 Glasshouse Yard, London EC1A 4JS
Tel: 020 7490 8818
Helpline: 0808 808 7777 (Mon–Fri
10 a.m.–12 p.m. and 2–4 p.m.)
Email: info@ukcarers.org
Website: www.carersuk.demon.co.uk
Offers information and support to people caring
for relatives and friends. Can put carers in touch
with local sources of information and help via its
national network branches and support groups.

Cinnamon Trust
Foundry House, Foundry Square, Hayle,
Cornwall TR27 4HE
Tel: 01736 757900
Email: admin@cinnamon.org.uk
Website: www.cinnamon.co.uk
The only specialist national charity for people in
their last years and their much loved companion
animals. A network of 3700 volunteers 'hold
hands' with owners to provide dog walking
and fostering for pets whilst their owners are in
hospital.

Citizens Advice Bureaux
Free impartial, confidential advice about death bereavement, financial and other matters. See your local phone book.

Counsel and Care
Twyman House, 16 Bonny Street,
London NW1 9PG
Helpline: 0845 300 7585 (Mon–Fri 10–12 a.m. and 2–4 p.m.)
Counsel and Care offer a comprehensive advice and information service for older people, their families and professionals. This service is free and confidential. It has a database of private home care agencies and benefits. Counsel and Care can provide some assistance to needy elderly people. It publishes information sheets on various topics.

Crossroads
10 Regent Place, Rugby,
Warwickshire CV21 2PN
Tel: 01788 573653
Crossroads aims to support carers and has a network of 207 care attendant schemes throughout the UK. They provide trained carers who take over and allow the regular carer to have a break. Contact the above number for further information and a list of local schemes. They also have an information pack.

The Disabled Living Foundation
380 Harrow Road, London W9 2HU
Tel: 020 7432 8009
Helpline: 0845 130 9177 (Mon–Fri 1–4 p.m.)

Gives practical, up-to-date, unbiased information and advice on all aspects of disability, especially equipment and problems of daily living. Provides displays and demonstrations of equipment. Also produces a wide range of publications including a comprehensive handbook of equipment. Visitors are welcome by appointment. Also provides a letter enquiry service.

Exit—The Voluntary Euthanasia Society of Scotland
17 Hart Street, Edinburgh EH1 3RN
Tel: 0131 556 4404
Email: exit@euthanasia.org
Website: www.euthanasia.org
The society supplies information and publications about all aspects of euthanasia.

Guide for Life
Wellington House, 28–32 Wellington Road, St John's Wood,
London NW8 9SP
Tel: 020 7483 9170
Email: webmaster@guideforlife.com
Website: www.guideforlife.com
An online network for people affected by illness, ageing, dying and bereavement in the UK and those who care for them. Offering impartial practical advice, support, information, service and products.

Holiday Care Service
2 Old Bank Chambers, Station Road, Horley, Surrey RH6 9HW
Tel: 01293 774 535

The Holiday Care Service is the UK's central resource for holiday information and support for disabled and disadvantaged people. There is no charge for this service. They also run a reservation service offering greatly discounted rates.

Hospice Information
St Christopher's Hospice,
51–59 Lawrie Park Road,
London SE26 6DZ
Tel: 0870 903 3903
Email: info@hospiceinformation.info
Website: www.hospiceinformation.info
Hospice Information provides an enquiry service about hospice and palliative care, including travel and holiday information for patients and carers. Publications include directories (both for the UK and the Republic of Ireland and international) of hospice and palliative care. The UK directory is free of charge but please send a large envelope with a £1 stamp. For details of local services please contact them directly.

Memory Store
Barnardo's Childcare Publications, Barnardo's Trading Estate, Paycocke Road, Basildon, Essex SS14 3DR
Tel: 01268 520 224
The Memory Store provides a practical way of bringing together important information for children who are losing contact with their parents. Orginally developed for families affected by HIV it can be used in many other situations such as adoption, marriage break-up or other illness.

Natural Death Centre
20 Heber Road,
London NW2 6AA
Tel: 020 8208 2853
This is an educational charity that aims to help
people wanting a natural low-tech death for which
they are spiritually and emotionally prepared.
They produce the *New Natural Death Handbook*
and their own living will. They give information
on woodland burial, biodegradable coffins, family-
organized and inexpensive funerals.

NHS Direct
Helpline: 0845 4647
Confidential twenty-four-hour helpline which
people can ring for advice and information on any
health concern or issue. Calls are answered by
experienced nurses and health information advis-
ers. They can provide information on a range of
issues including medical conditions, support groups
and health services in your area.

Rainbow Trust
Rainbow House,
47 Eastwick Drive,
Great Bookham,
Leatherhead, Surrey KT23 3PU
Tel: 01372 453 309 or 01372 363 438 (admin)
Supports and cares for children with life-threaten-
ing or terminal illness and their families. Provides
physical and emotional support either at home or
in Rainbow House, a respite haven that enables
sick children to enjoy a break with their parents,
brothers and sisters.

Red Cross Medical Loans Service
See your local phone book for details. Branches
can supply equipment such as wheelchairs, commodes, etc. for short-term loan.

Triscope
The Courtyard,
Evelyn Road, London W4 5JL
Tel: 0208 580 7021
A travel and transport information service for
disabled and elderly people. The telephone-based
service is available free of charge to disabled and
elderly people and those who care for them. Help
can be given on planning journeys, whatever the
distance, and with answers to a whole range of
travel-related questions.

Urostomy Association
'Buckland', Beaumont Park,
Danebury, Essex CM3 4DE
Tel: 01245 224 294
Assists patients before and after surgery with counselling on appliances, housing, work situations or
marital problems. Helps them to resume as full a
life as possible with confidence. Branch meetings
held. Can also arrange hospital and home visits by
former patients on request.

The Voluntary Euthanasia Society (UK)
13 Prince of Wales Terrace,
London W8 5PG
Tel: 020 7937 7770
Email: info@ves.org.uk
The society provides information on all aspects of
euthanasia. It also supplies its own living will.

Organizations for patients with cancer

Breast Cancer Care
Kiln House, 210 New Kings Road,
London SW6 4NZ
Tel: 020 7384 2984
Helpline: 0808 800 6000 (Mon–Fri 10 a.m.–5 p.m.;
Sat 10 a.m.–2 p.m.)
Email: bcc@breastcancercare.org.uk
Provides free help, information and support to women and men with breast cancer or other breast-related problems, as well as to their families, partners and friends.

Bristol Cancer Help Centre
See p. 236.

Cancer BACUP
3 Bath Place, Rivington Street,
London EC2A 3JR
Tel: 020 7696 9003
Helpline: 0808 800 1234 (Mon–Fri 9 a.m.–7 p.m.)
Email: info@cancerbacup.org
Trained cancer nurses provide information, emotional support and practical advice by telephone, letter or email for patients with cancer and their families and friends.

The Cancer Care Society (CARE)
Jane Scarth House, 39 The Hundred, Romsey,
Hampshire, SO51 8GE
Tel: 01794 830374
Emotional support and practical advice for anyone whose life has been affected by cancer: patients, carers, family, friends. Mainly telephone counselling.

It has a national linkline for people so that they can get support from others who have experienced similar symptoms or worries. Also drop-in centres in Portsmouth and South Wales.

Cancer Relief Macmillan Fund
89 Albert Embankment, London SE1 7UQ
Tel: 020 7840 7840
9 Castle Terrace, Edinburgh EH1 2DP
Tel: 0131 229 3276
Information about Macmillan units for inpatients, day care and Macmillan nurses. Ring to find out if help is available in your area. Patient grant applications to the Macmillan Fund should be made via community, hospital and hospice nurses, social workers and other care professionals.

Cancerlink
11–21 Northdown Street,
London N1 9BN
Tel: 020 7833 2818
Provides emotional support and information over the telephone on all aspects of cancer, and the opportunity to link with other people living with cancer. Resource for over 700 self-help and support groups across the UK.

Complementary Cancer Care Programme
See p. 237.

Macmillan Information Line
89 Albert Embankment,
London SE1 7UQ
Helpline: 0845 601 6161 (Mon–Fri
9.30 a.m–7.30 p.m.)
Email: information_line@macmillan.org.uk

Telephone information service about Macmillan services and activities as well as other available support organizations.

Marie Curie Cancer Care
89 Albert Embankment, London SEI 7TP
Tel: 020 7599 7777
There are ten Marie Curie centres throughout the country and nine of these provide a home care service. A day and night nursing service at home is available in most health authorities. The organization has a welfare grant scheme. Apply initially through the community nursing services (district nurses) for nursing care, but you can ring the above number for further details.

Sargent Cancer Care for Children
Griffin House, 161 Hammersmith Road,
London W6 8SG
Tel: 020 8752 2800
Can provide cash grants for parents of children aged up to twenty-one with cancer, to help with clothing, equipment, travel, fuel bills, etc. Apply through a hospital social worker or ring the fund and ask for advice on other ways to apply, such as through your GP.

Sue Ryder Care
Healthcare Services, Sue Ryder Care, PO Box 5044, Ashby de la Zouch,
Leicestershire LE65 1ZP
Tel: 01332 694800
Website: www.suerydercare.org
Seven homes in England that specialize in cancer care. Visiting nurses care for patients in their own

homes. Usually contacted via your community nursing team or other health professionals but for further details ring the above number.

Tak Tent
Cancer Support Organization, Flat 5,
30 Shelly Court, Gartnavel,
Gloucestershire G12 0YN
Tel: 0141 211 0122
Website: www.taktent.org.uk
Gives emotional support and information on cancers and treatments to patients, family, friends and medical staff, either over the phone or at the resource centre in a private one-to-one setting. Has support groups throughout Scotland, including one for 16–25 year olds.

Tenovus Cancer Information Centre
College Buildings, Courtenay Road, Splott,
Cardiff CF1 1SA
Tel: 029 2049 7700
An information, support and counselling service for people with cancer and their families. The cancer helpline is manned by trained cancer nurses and there is also a social worker and counseller available to talk to you. Small financial grants are available. There is a library for the use of patients or professionals. Contact by phone or letter.

Other specific organizations

If you suffer from a disease that is not listed below ask your GP or consultant if there is a charity that might help you. Alternatively ask at your library, who have access to a list of all British charities, or ring NHS Direct on 0845 4647.

Motor Neurone Disease Association
PO Box 246, Northampton NN1 2PR
Tel: 01604 250505 or 01604 22269
(twenty-four-hour service)
Helpline: 0845 300 0336
Email: enquiries@mndassociation.org
Website: www.mndassociation.org
Produces useful factsheets for sufferers and carers, as well as a professional advice pack. Their care service can help with equipment loans for sufferers. Regional care advisors who have paramedical backgrounds can give advice or education on care. Financial aid for sufferers and a social and health-care pack for professionals are also available. One of the few societies to provide information specifically on terminal care.

Multiple Sclerosis Society
MS National Centre,
372 Edgware Road,
London NW2 6ND
Tel: 020 8438 0700
Helpline: 0808 800 8000
Email: info@mssociety.org.uk
Website: www.mssociety.org.uk
Offers information to people with MS, their friends, carers and family. Financial assistance and welfare services are available. There are over 360 local branches.

National AIDS Helpline
Freephone 0800 567 123

For anyone requiring information and advice on AIDS and HIV infection. The helpline will give you information about both national and local services. It also offers a telephone counselling service.

The Naz Project (London)
Pallingswick House, 241 King Street,
London W6 9LP
Tel: 020 8741 1879
Email: naz@naz.org.uk
Sexual health and HIV and AIDS education, prevention and support services for the South Asian, Middle Eastern and North African communities. Support groups for people affected and for their carers.

Parkinson's Disease Society
215 Vauxhall Bridge Road, London SW1V 1EJ
Tel: 020 7931 8080
Helpline: 0808 800 0303
(Mon–Fri 9.30 a.m.– 5.30 p.m.)
Email: enquiries@parkinsons.org.uk
Helps all people with Parkinson's disease and their families. The society provides welfare information, education and field services. There are 255 local branches. You can find these listed in your local phone book.

The Stroke Association
123–127 Whitecross Street,
London EC1Y 8JJ
Tel: 020 7566 0300
Helpline: 0845 303 3100
Email: stroke@stroke.org.uk
Website: www.stroke.org.uk

Local information and support services are listed in the local phone book. The Stroke Association has information centres and care groups, including Stroke Clubs around the country. It publishes information for both patients and their carers.

The Terrence Higgins Trust Lighthouse
52–54 Grays Inn Road,
London WC1X 8JU
Tel: 020 7831 0330
Helpline: 0171 242 1010
(daily 12 a.m–10 p.m.)
Email: info@tht.org.uk
Website: www.tht.org.uk
Provides information, advice and help to all those concerned about AIDS and HIV infection. Practical help includes 'buddies' for people with AIDS in the London area; welfare, housing and legal advice; counselling; and support groups.

Complementary medicine

The Bristol Cancer Help Centre
Grove House, Cornwallis Grove, Clifton,
Bristol BS8 4PG
Tel: 0117 980 9500
Helpline: 0117 980 9505
Email: info@bristolcancerhelp.org
Website: www.bristolcancerhelp.org
Offers a holistic healing programme (to complement medical treatment) including relaxation, counselling, healing, nutrition, visualization and meditation. Patients can attend for a residential two- or five-day course.

The British Holistic Medical Association
Tel: 01273 725951
Email: bhma@bhma.org
Website: www.bhma.org
Publications include self-help tapes on breathing, relaxation, meditation, imagery and coping with pain.

Complementary Cancer Care Programme
The Royal London Homeopathic Hospital NHS Trust, Great Ormond Street,
London WC1N 3HR
Tel: 020 7837 8833 ext 7239/7240
(contact Dr S. Kassab)
Offers a programme of homeopathy and other complementary therapies to support well-being and quality of life, which may be used in conjunction with conventional cancer treatments.

Bereavement services

The Compassionate Friends
53 North Street, Bristol BS3 1EN
Tel: 0117 966 5202
Helpline: 0117 953 9639
(daily 9.30 a.m.–10.30 p.m.)
Email: info@tcf.org.uk
Website: www.tcf.org.uk
A nationwide organization offering support and friendship to bereaved parents and their families after the death of a child, of any age and due to any cause. There are also support groups for parents having lost a child through suicide or murder.

CRUSE
CRUSE Bereavement Care,
Cruse House, 126 Sheen Road,
Richmond, Surrey TW9 1UR
Helpline: 0870 167 1677
Offers free bereavement counselling, support and information to anyone bereaved by death. The society has an extensive publications list along with useful leaflets, and offers social contacts as well as specialist services to various bereaved groups.

Lesbian and Gay Bereavement Project
1a Waterlow Road,
London N19 5NJ
Tel: 020 8281 5297
Helpline: 020 8455 8894
(Mon–Fri 7–10.30 p.m.)
Email: lgbp@lgbp.freeserve.co.uk
Website: www.members.aol.com/lgbp
Offers advice, support and counselling to bereaved gay men and lesbians, their families and friends.

National Association of Bereavement Services
2nd floor, 4 Pinchin Street, London E1 1SA
Tel: 020 7709 0505
Helpline: 020 7709 9090
This very useful association has a comprehensive nationwide directory of bereavement and loss services and can help put you in touch with the right local groups for you. It covers diverse groups offering support for people of different religions, races, sexuality and ages, and for different kinds of illness or loss. It is staffed by bereavement counsellors.

Winston's Wish
Clara Burgess Centre, Gloucester Royal Hospital,
Great Western Road,
Gloucester GL1 3NN
Tel: 01452 394377
Helpline: 0845 203 0405
Email: info@winstonswish.org.uk
Website: www. winstonswish.org.uk
Winston's Wish, a grief support programme,
provides a range of services for bereaved children
and their families.

Appendix 4:
Recommended Reading

Facing Death, Averil Stedford. William Heinemann Medical Books, London, 1984.

The *New Natural Death Handbook*, Nicholas Albery, Stephanie Wienrich. RIDER Books, London, 2000.

Dancing with Mister D. Notes on Life and Death, Bert Keizer. Black Swan Press, Grove, Oxon, 1995.

All in the End is Harvest, an Anthology for Those who Grieve, Agnes Whitaker. Darton, Longman and Todd, London, 1984.

What to do After a Death, Department of Social Security.
Help When Someone Dies, Department of Social Security. Both of these comprehensive and helpful leaflets are available from your local DSS office or from DSS Leaflets Unit, PO Box 21, Stanmore, Middlesex HAY 1AY.

Arranging a Funeral (factsheet), Age Concern. Write or telephone for a free leaflet (See p. 223.)

Funerals, a Guide, James Bentley, Andrew Best and Jackie Hunt. Hodder and Stoughton, London, 1994.

Funerals Without God: a Practical Guide to Non-Religious Funerals, Jane Wynne Willson. Available from the British Humanist Association, 47 Theobald's Road, London WC1X 8SP, telephone 020 7430 0908.

Before We say Goodbye: Preparing for a Good Death, Ray Simpson. Harper Collins, London, 2001.

Index

acceptance 115–16
acupuncture 16
advance directives, *see* living
  wills
AGE Concern 61, 82, 128,
  223
AIDS/HIV
  'buddies' 61
  cannabis benefits in 203
  district nurse's role 37
  hospices 95, 99
  *Living Proof: Courage in
    the Face of AIDS* (Jones) 30,
    117
  loss of appetite 188
  National AIDS Helpline 12,
    234–5
  parents with 122–3
  sexuality 141
  specialist hospitals 77
  The Terrence Higgins Trust
    Lighthouse 20, 89, 130, 236
alcohol 92, 169
anger 1–2, 112–13, 116
  carer's 145–6
  with medical staff 64
  unexpressed 7
antidepressant drugs 163, 165,
  166, 167
  side effects 167, 170
antisickness drugs 186, 189
anxiety
  carer's 147–52
  patient's 160–3
    causing breathlessness 190–1
anxiolytics 163
  see also diazepam (Valium);
    nabilone
appetite loss 188–90
appetite stimulants 190
aromatherapy 18–19, 163
aspirin 178

assessment
  needs 21–2
  pain 176–8
attendance allowance 219

bargaining 113–14, 116
bed (pressure) sores 171–4
bereavement support services
  55–6, 145, 237–9
birth plans 134
bone cancer 185, 199
brain tumours 199–200
breaking bad news
  doctors 6–7, 87–8
  to children 10–11
  to family and friends 9–10
breast cancer 139–40
breathing difficulties 150, 190–4,
  194
  self-help 193
  treatment 191–3
Bristol Cancer Help Centre
  17–18, 230, 236
British Association for
  Counselling and Psychotherapy
  20, 223
British Colostomy Association
  140, 171, 224
British Medical Association 130

cancer 4–5
  bone 185, 199
  brain 199–200
  breast 139–40
  Bristol Cancer Help Centre
    17–18, 230, 236
  cannabis benefits in 203
  district nurse's role 37
  information sources 12, 13,
    230–3

cancer (*cont.*)
  loss of appetite 188
  organizations 230–3
  specialist hospitals 77
  specialists 45, 52
  see also hospices
CancerLink 12, 231
Cancer Relief Macmillan
  Fund 162, 221–2, 231
cannabis 92, 203–4
  see also nabilone
care homes, *see* nursing and
  residential homes
carer(s)
  adapting to role 25–6
  alleviating burden of 74–5, 93–4
  anger 145–6
  anxiety 147–52
  attitudes to patient's
    depression 114–15
  denial 111–12
  elderly 70–1
  exhaustion 146–7
  good feelings 143–4
  guilt 93
  intuition 3–4
  needs 42, 90
  –patient relationships 75–6,
    136–9
  practical concerns 152–6
  selfish feelings 146–7
  –staff relationships 88–90
  see also family
Carers National Association
  26, 149, 224
catheterization 173, 196
chaplains, *see* ministers of the
  church
charities 24–5, 221–2
chemists 60–1
chest infections 8, 192–3, 199
Cheyne–Stokes breathing 150,
  194
children
  attitudes to staff 86
  breaking bad news to 10–11

dependent 120–1, 141–2
  in home of elderly patient
    152–3
  hospices for 95, 99
  leaving gifts for 122–3
chiropractors 16
Christianity 133, 135
  ethos of hospices 104
  Roman Catholics 132
  see also ministers of the church
chronic illness 7–8, 70–1
Church Council 61
colostomies 140, 170–1, 224
commodes 195
communication
  between professionals 32–3,
    34, 36–7, 61–3
  between staff and carers 89–90
  with confused patients 201–2
  poor 61–3
Community Care Act (1993) 21,
  30, 90
community hospitals 78–9
community nurses, *see* district
  nurses
Compassionate Friends 120,
  237
complementary therapy 15–19
  in hospices 104
  in hospitals 91
  organizations 236–7
  pain relief 177
condoms 140, 141
confidentiality 37, 90
confusion 198–203
  drug-induced 181, 199
constipation 167–71
  causes 181, 198, 199
consultants 77, 78, 87
co-proxamol 170, 178
coroners 217
counselling 19–20, 166–7
creams 196
creativity 18
Crossroads 149, 154, 225
CRUSE 145, 238

Dancing with Mr D (Kaiser) 133, 241
day centres 154
day hospices 98–9
death
  approaching 3–6
  'good' 1, 69, 70
  moment of 149–50, 209–14
  what to do after 150–2, 217–18
death (medical) certificate 151, 217
decision-making
  in hospices 103
  regarding treatment 13–14
denial 85, 109–12
  of symptoms 158
dentures 174, 189
dependents, *see* children; family; parents, dependent; spouses (partners)
depression 114–15, 116, 166–7
dexamethasone 164
diagnosis 4–5, 44–5
  discussing with GP 42, 43
diamorphine 45
  see also morphine
diaries 158
diazepam (Valium) 192
diet, *see* food
dieticians 32–3
dignity 84
disability living allowance 219–20
Disabled Living Foundation 25, 225–6
distress 208–9
district general hospitals 77
district nurses 33–4
  how to contact 36–8
    after patient's death 150
  individual strengths and weaknesses 38
  referral to specialist nurses 55, 57
  roles 35–6, 37
  seeking advice from 155

team members 34–5
treatment of constipation 170
doctors
  approaches to decision-making 14
  attitudes to complementary therapy 16–17
  attitudes to euthanasia 132
  breaking bad news 6–7, 87–8
  consultants 77, 78, 87
  hospice 58, 184–5
  responses to 'how long have I got?' 7–8
  specialists 58
  uncaring 64–5
  see also general practitioners (GPs)
drinking 169, 187
  alcohol 92, 169
drowsiness 181
dry lips 175
dry mouth 181
  see also mouth care
Durogesic, *see* fentanyl
Dying Process, The (Lawton) 103–4

elderly carers 70–1
elderly patients
  AGE Concern 61, 82, 128, 223
  confusion 199
  food for 189
  home care workers 59
  home visits by geriatrician 58
  residential and nursing homes 80–2
email groups 13
emergency admission to hospital 73–4
emotional pain 19
emotional support
  by GPs 45–6
  by home care nurses 53
  in hospital 72
empathy 54

Index

enemas 170
euthanasia 130, 131–3, 226, 229
exercise 165, 169
exhaustion, carer's 146–7
Exit 133, 226
extended families 121–2

false hope 16–17
family
  breaking bad news to 9–10
  estrangements 125
  extended 121–2
  GP consultations with 42
  hospice philosophy 102
  needs 88
  types 89
  see also carer(s); children;
    parents, dependent; spouses
    (partners)
fentanyl (Durogesic) 169, 184
  patches 184
financial assistance 23–4, 162,
  219–22
financial planning 119, 134
food
  attractively presented 189
  as complementary therapy 18
  for elderly 189
  high-fibre 168–9
  hospital 91
  liquid supplements 189–90
  nausea-inducing 186–7
friends
  breaking bad news to 9–10
  GP consultations with 42
funeral directors (undertakers)
  151, 217, 218
funerals 134–6
  alternative 136, 151–2, 218

general practitioners (GPs)
  39–51
  beds in community hospitals 78
  changing 66

  reasons for 62–3, 64, 65
  choice of 39–40
  contacting after patient's death
    150–1, 217
  co-operatives 40–1
  home care 31–3, 39–51
  home visits 40, 42–3, 44
  individual strengths and
    weaknesses 45–6
  letting you down 63–4
  nursing homes 81
  out of hours calls 40–1
  referral
    to hospice 106
    to hospital 105
  roles 42–5, 55
  who will not ask for help
    65–6
  see also doctors
geriatricians 58
gifts, leaving 122–5
goodbyes 85–6, 150, 151,
  206–8
'good death' 1, 69, 70
good feelings
  carer's 143–4
  see also positive experiences

healing 16
health care assistants,
  district 35
hearing 202–3
heel protectors (Tubipads) 172
HIV, see AIDS/HIV
holistic approach
  hospices 97, 102
  see also complementary
    therapy
home care
  community team members
    30–51
  specialists involved in 51–61
  vs hospital care 26–7, 29–30,
    31, 72–6
  what can go wrong 61–6

home care specialist (Macmillan)
nurses 31, 52–6
how to contact 54–5
responses to 54
roles 52–4
home care workers 59
homeopaths 16
home responsibilities
protection 220
home visits
by GPs 40, 42–3, 44
by specialist doctors 58
hope 8–9, 116
false 16–17
through self-help techniques 18
hospice doctors 58, 184–5
Hospice Information Service
227
hospices 94–106
arranging admission to 53–4
at home 56
attitudes to admission 99–101
complementary therapy
available in 18–19
control of pain 73
control of symptoms 31
day 98–9
holistic approach 97, 102
and palliative care units 98
reasons for admission 101–2
reasons for choosing 102–5
referral to 106
specialist 99
staff 102–3, 104–5
hospital discharge letter 42, 43
hospitals 68–94
choosing 76–7, 82–3, 92–4
exacerbation of confusion 202
patient needs 90–2
patient—patient relationships
84–6, 160
patient—staff relationships
86–8
referrals to 105–6
side rooms 79, 83
staff—carer relationships 88–90

types 76–82
vs home care 26–7, 29–30, 31,
72–6
ward sisters 106, 155
wards, organization and
structure 83

iliostomies 170
incontinence 194–7
bowel 197–8
incontinence nurse
specialists 57, 140
incontinence pads 173, 195
disposal 197
infections
chest 8, 192–3, 199
urinary 194, 196, 199
information sources 11–13,
223–39
internet 13
intestacy 127–8
intuition 3–4
invalid care allowance 220
isolation 72, 84–5

key workers 32–3, 39, 55
Kubler-Ross, Elizabeth 108,
113

last days
distress 208–9
goodbyes 85–6, 150, 151,
206–8
see also death
laundry 196–7
laxatives 169, 170
leaving gifts 122–5
legal matters 127–33
letting go 214–15
*Living Proof: Courage in the Face
of AIDS* (Jones) 30, 117
living wills 129–31
loneliness, *see* isolation

Index

loss
  of appetite 188–90
  of bladder/bowel control, *see*
    incontinence
  of freedom 92
  of income and status 138
  of weight 174, 188
love affairs 126–7

Macmillan Fund 162, 221–2,
  231
Macmillan nurses, *see* home
  care specialist (Macmillan)
  nurses
Marie Curie Foundation 57, 155,
  232
Marie Curie nurses 57, 154.
massage 18–19, 146, 163, 177
  shiatsu 16
mattresses 165, 172, 196
medical (death) certificate 151,
  217
meditation 18, 177
memory
  long-term 200–1
  short-term 202
'memory store' 122–3, 227
ministers of the church 60
  hospice 32–3
  hospital 60, 76
morphine 45
  for breathlessness 192
  how to take 181–2
  injections 183–4
  mechanism of action 180
  'myth' 178–80
  oral 178
    MST 182
  regular review 182–3
  side effects 169, 179, 180–1
morphine suphate continuous
  (MST) 182
motor neurone disease 95,
  191

Motor Neurone Disease
  Association 12, 24, 191, 234
mouth care 174–5, 181
moving house 62–3
multidisciplinary meetings 33
multiple sclerosis 7–8, 95, 203–4
Multiple Sclerosis Society 12,
  234
Muslims 4, 104

nabilone 192
National AIDS Helpline 12,
  234–5
National Association of
  Bereavement Services 145, 238
National Care Standards
  Commission 82
Natural Death Centre 136, 228
natural energy 15–16, 19
nausea and vomiting 181,
  185–8
nebulizers 192
needs
  carer's 42, 90
  family 88
  patient's
    assessment 21–2
    in hospital 90–2
New Natural Death Handbook,
  The (Albery) 136, 152, 218,
  241
NHS Direct 12, 41, 228
night nurses 57–8, 153–4
  district nursing team 35
nitrazepam 165
non-cancer conditions 5–6, 95
  see also specific conditions
nurses
  in community hospitals 78, 79
  letting you down 63–4
  in private hospitals 79
  see also specific roles
nursing and residential homes
  80–1

nursing sisters
 district 34–5
 hospital 106, 155

occupational therapists 22, 59
opioids, *see* co-proxamol;
 morphine
oral candidiasis (thrush) 174–5,
 189
organ donation 217–18
osteopaths 16
out of hours calls, GPs 40–1
oxygen 191–2, 199

pain 175–85
 acute and chronic 176
 assessment 176–8
 descriptions of 176
 emotional 19
pain clinics 184–5
pain control 45, 177–85
 aim of treatment 175–6
 hospital/hospice admission for
  73, 92–3
 inadequate, causing
  sleeplessness 165
 'ladder' 177–8
 special 184–5
palliative care 96–8
 specialists 58, 76–7
 see also home care specialist
  (Macmillan) nurses;
  hospices
paracetamol 178
parents, dependent 120
Parkinson's Disease Society 12,
 24, 235
partners (spouses) 119
patient(s)
 –carer relationships 75–6,
  136–9
 comparing treatments 12
 participation 14, 16

–patient relationships 84–6, 160
responses to home care nurses 54
–staff relationships 63, 86–8
penile sheaths 195–6
personality clashes 63
pets 91, 162
pharmacists 60–1
photographic records 123–5
plastic mattresses 196
pneumonia 192–3
position
 changing 172
 upright 193
positive experiences 116–18
 see also good feelings, carer's
Potter, Dennis 117–18
power of attorney 128–9
pregnant mothers 134
prescriptions, free 221
pressure (bed) sores 171–4
pressure mattresses 165
priests, *see* ministers of the
 church
privacy, lack of 84, 90
private hospitals 79–80
private nurses 154
psychologists 76
psychotherapy 167

referrals
 to counsellor/psychotherapist
  20, 167
 to home care nurses 54–5
 to hospice 106
 to hospital 105–6
 to pain specialist 185
 to specialist nurses 57
 to specialist palliative care
  team 77
relationships 136–9
 carer—staff 88–90
 love affairs 126–7
 sexuality 139–41
 see also patient(s)

relaxation 18, 146, 177
religion, *see* Christianity;
  ministers of the church;
  Muslims
residential and nursing
  homes 80–1
respite care 94, 154–5
role changes 137–9
Roman Catholics 132

Saunders, Dame Cicely 96
second opinions 14–15
secrets 126–7
sedatives 163
self-help 18
  breathing difficulties 193
  groups 24–5
selfish feelings, carer's 146–7
self-referral 106
self-responsibility 19
sexuality 139–41
sheepskin 172
shiatsu massage 16
sight 202–3
sleeping tablets 164, 165
sleeplessness 163–6
smells, preventing 196–7
smoking 91–2
social services 21–3, 24, 154
social workers 22, 59, 82
specialist doctors 58
specialist hospices 99
specialist hospitals 77
specialist nurses 56–8
  palliative care 32–3, 76
specialist palliative care
  teams 76–7
Spenco cushions and
  mattresses 172
spiritual support, *see* ministers of
  the church
spouses (partners) 119
  see also carer(s)
sputum 193

staff
  hospice 102–3, 104–5
  hospital 88–90
staff nurses, district 35
'stages' of dying 108–16
statutory benefits 219–22
statutory services 21–3
stoma care specialists 57,
  170–1
Stroke Association 235–6
strokes 68–9, 70, 200
student nurses 86
suicide 114, 133
suppositories 170
symptom control 31
  by GPS 44–5
  by nurses 53, 57
  hospital/hospice admission
    for 73, 92–3
  in nursing homes 81
symptoms
  denial 158
  influences on 159–60
  talking about 157–60
syringe drivers 45, 183–4
  antisickness drugs via 186

Tak Tent 12, 20, 233
Tegaderm 173
temazepam 165
temperature in hospitals 91
Terrence Higgins Trust
  Lighthouse, The 20, 89,
  130, 236
tests 45
thrush (oral candidiasis) 174–5,
  189
Tubipads (heel protectors) 172

uncaring doctors 64–5
undertakers, *see* funeral
  directors
unemployment 138

unfinished business 125–7
urinals 195
urinary infections 194, 196, 199

Valium (diazepam) 192
visitors 83, 153, 155
visualization 18
Voluntary Euthanasia Society
  130, 133, 229
voluntary organizations 20, 61,
  154
vomiting, *see* nausea and
  vomiting

wandering 203
ward cleaners 86
weight loss 174, 188
wills 127–8
  living 129–31

yoga 146, 177
young patients 2

Zomorph (MST) 182